SpringerBriefs in Sociology

Series editor

Robert J. Johnson, University of Miami, Coral Gables, FL, USA

More information about this series at http://www.springer.com/series/10410

Robert J. Johnson · R. Jay Turner · Bruce G. Link
Editors

Sociology of Mental Health

Selected Topics from Forty Years
1970s–2010s

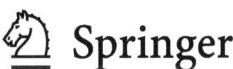 Springer

Editors
Robert J. Johnson
Department of Sociology
University of Miami
Coral Gables, FL
USA

Bruce G. Link
Columbia University
New York, NY
USA

R. Jay Turner
Department of Sociology
Vanderbilt University
Nashville, TN
USA

ISSN 2212-6368   ISSN 2212-6376   (electronic)
ISBN 978-3-319-07796-3   ISBN 978-3-319-07797-0   (eBook)
DOI 10.1007/978-3-319-07797-0

Library of Congress Control Number: 2014947663

Springer Cham Heidelberg New York Dordrecht London

© The Author(s) 2014
This work is subject to copyright. All rights are reserved by the Publisher, whether the whole or part of the material is concerned, specifically the rights of translation, reprinting, reuse of illustrations, recitation, broadcasting, reproduction on microfilms or in any other physical way, and transmission or information storage and retrieval, electronic adaptation, computer software, or by similar or dissimilar methodology now known or hereafter developed. Exempted from this legal reservation are brief excerpts in connection with reviews or scholarly analysis or material supplied specifically for the purpose of being entered and executed on a computer system, for exclusive use by the purchaser of the work. Duplication of this publication or parts thereof is permitted only under the provisions of the Copyright Law of the Publisher's location, in its current version, and permission for use must always be obtained from Springer. Permissions for use may be obtained through RightsLink at the Copyright Clearance Center. Violations are liable to prosecution under the respective Copyright Law.
The use of general descriptive names, registered names, trademarks, service marks, etc. in this publication does not imply, even in the absence of a specific statement, that such names are exempt from the relevant protective laws and regulations and therefore free for general use.
While the advice and information in this book are believed to be true and accurate at the date of publication, neither the authors nor the editors nor the publisher can accept any legal responsibility for any errors or omissions that may be made. The publisher makes no warranty, express or implied, with respect to the material contained herein.

Printed on acid-free paper

Springer is part of Springer Science+Business Media (www.springer.com)

Preface

This volume commemorates the 20th Anniversary of the American Sociological Association (ASA) Section on the Sociology of Mental Health. Jay Turner reminded us of this upcoming anniversary with a suggestion he made at end of the Section's business meeting during the ASA's annual meeting in Las Vegas in 2011. He suggested that something should be done to commemorate the event. I had just been installed as the incoming Chair of the section, and I assured the members in attendance that something would be done, but I was unsure just what that would be.

About one month later, Bob Johnson sent an email to me suggesting that the Section anniversary be commemorated with a volume of papers reviewing progress in mental health sociology and laying out critical research problems for the future. The volume would be sponsored by the Section, and all remuneration would be contributed to the Section. I agreed that it was a great idea. With guidance from Karen Edwards, Director of Publications for ASA, and approval from the Section Publications Committee, we developed a proposal for the ASA Publications Committee that was approved in early December 2011. Bob recruited two additional editors, Jay Turner and Bruce Link, two sociologists who are responsible for much of the progress in the sociology of mental health over the past 40 years.

The chapters in the current volume document select theoretical transformations and refinements of the field from the issues that animated our studies in the 1970s and 1980s to a new set of problems and challenges. The sociology of mental health was founded by scholars interested in showing how social integration, urban life, and social class were related to psychological problems. Chapters in this volume show how these fairly straightforward issues have been transformed into a set of questions about complex processes linking stress, social relationships and support, neighborhoods, societal reactions and other factors to mental health, mental disorder and other outcomes. One of the most energetic debates in sociology in the last 45 years was between advocates of the labeling theory of mental illness and those supporting a psychiatric perspective. As is clear from the chapters in the present volume on stigma, on stress, and on recovery from mental illness, this debate resulted in a considerable refinement of the issues, and created a new set of research problems. Another controversial issue in the 1970s was whether and how gender was related to mental health and illness. As can be seen by the chapter on gender and marital status in the present volume, this issue too has been transformed from relatively simple questions about sex roles and marital roles into ones involving social identities, varying distress styles, sociocultural and socioeconomic contexts, multiple dimensions of mental health, the nature of intimate relationships, and other factors.

As a group, this set of papers not only traces significant changes in the sociology of mental health, but also testifies to the health of the field itself and to the wisdom of the section founders. Along with the recent establishment of the section journal, *Society and Mental Health*, and the publication of the second editions of two handbooks on the sociology of mental health (Scheid and Brown 2010; Aneshensel et al. 2013), this volume shows that there are many questions to answer, but there is progress to be had, and there are ways to move forward.

Michael Hughes

References

Aneshensel, C. S., Phelan, J. C., & Bierman, A. (2013). *A Handbook for the Study of Mental Health* (2nd ed.). New York: Springer.

Scheid, T. L., & Brown, T. N. (2010). *A Handbook for the Study of Mental Health* (2nd ed.). New York: Cambridge University Press.

Contents

1 **Social Relationships and Social Support**.................... 1
  R. Jay Turner, J. Blake Turner and William Beardall Hale

2 **Twenty Years of the Sociology of Mental Health:
  The Continued Significance of Gender and Marital
  Status for Emotional Well-Being**............................. 21
  Robin W. Simon

3 **The Stress Process: Its Origins, Evolution, and Future**............ 53
  Carol S. Aneshensel and Uchechi A. Mitchell

4 **Mental Illness Stigma and the Sociology of Mental Health**.......... 75
  Bruce G. Link and Jo C. Phelan

5 **The Neighborhood and Mental Life: Past, Present,
  and Future Sociological Directions in Studying
  Community Context and Mental Health**....................... 101
  Richard M. Carpiano

6 **Everything Old Is New Again: Recovery and Serious Mental Illness**... 125
  Dennis P. Watson, Anne McCranie and Eric R. Wright

7 **Impact of Mental Health Research in Sociology:
  Nearly Four Decades of Scholarship (1975–2011)**................. 141
  Robert J. Johnson

Introduction

It was tempting at first to propose that we name this monograph "Score I for the Section on the Sociology of Mental Health." The title would intend to suggest both that the section had just past its first 20 year mark and that the research on the sociology of mental health had scored big by being particularly productive over those 20 years. The chapters in this monograph, as you will discover, do in fact support both those initial observations. Perhaps, however, the title should have been "Score II for the Section of the Sociology of Mental Health" as it is not only just beginning a second 20 year period, but also because the apparent success during the 20 years prior had clearly provide a sense of the need and laid the foundation for its formation. Does one look back or forward? Not surprisingly, given such a choice, we quickly settled on the answer to provide a brief look at both.

Impetus for this Commemorative Monograph

The boom years in the sociology of mental health research (as Turner, Turner and Hale call them in this volume) began in the seventh decade of the last century peaking during the eighth decade for the first time attributable importantly (Johnson and Wolinsky 1990) but not wholly (Mechanic 1990) to the legacy of stress research and sustaining themselves over the course of the first score years subsequent to the foundation of the Section on the Sociology of Mental Health. An early consensus, even if settled but on only a couple of points (albeit a major ones), was that stress research broadly shared interests with many overlapping areas of mental health research in general and that to the extent we can rely on citations as an objective measure of impact, sociological journals that publish such areas of interest rank well compared to others commonly perceived to be prestigious in sociology generally. The questions of where this would lead us over the subsequent years would largely be addressed by the leaders and members of this section of the American Sociological Association that was just newly forming at that time.

The research continued as the years passed, and at the end of the business meeting of the Section on the Sociology of Mental Health (SSMH) in Las Vegas 2011, Jay Turner stood to remind the attendees that the 20th Anniversary of the section would be during the next meeting in Denver 2012. He suggested that something be done to commemorate that event. The incoming president of the section, Michael Hughes thanked him for the reminder and the meeting soon adjourned. At that meeting I was there to hear the reminder, and I also quite separate from that event agreed to launch a monograph series in sociology for Springer. As I prepared the announcement for monographs later that year, I remembered Jay's suggestion and dropped a note to Michael asking him if he thought a commemorative monograph on mental health research would be a fitting tribute.

The Commemorative Monograph Proposal

At the request of Michael Hughes, a proposal was prepared and submitted to the Sociology of Mental Health (SMH) council and Committee on Publications. The proposal to produce a commemorative monograph was intended to embody the spirit of the rise to prominence, the continuing success, and the promise members of the section find on the frontiers of research in mental health as the section moves into the future. The monograph was to be a brief, peer-reviewed monograph of article length manuscripts.

The introduction was proposed to provide both a broad retrospective of mental health research and introduce each manuscript for the reader. The topics of each selected manuscript were intended to be both retrospective and farsighted, (1) reviewing key findings in well-defined threads of research that potential new contributors to the field must understand in order to make independent advances and (2) providing insights for future directions that continue that thread or expand it into multi-threads of research.

A list of potential topics and contributors was developed and reviewed by the monograph editors. Manuscripts would be invited from authors based on solicited topics. They would be selected from members of the Section on Mental Health with a balance among key figures in the field, inaugural members of the section, and new promising scholars. Pairings of established and emerging scholars may be an effective means of achieving this goal.

Proceeds collected by the contributors from the publisher of this monograph will be committed to the section.

Origins of Sociology and the Sociology of Mental Health Research

At the core of American sociology is the concept of the "self." It is arguably the most fundamental concept to distinguish sociology from its sister disciplines, particularly psychology. Yet it is also the concept that bridges the disciplines in the interdisciplinary field of social psychology. And more importantly, it was borrowed from the very foundations of American psychology through the work of William James and his influence on the giants in the first school of American sociology at the University of Chicago. The "hidden self" was James' concept (1890) that he explored in an effort to understand mental illness, an understanding that eluded him in his own fields of scholarly training, medicine, and physiology. It was an understanding he sought not only in terms of the mental illness of others, but also in terms of his own struggles with depression and his lifelong commitment to promoting public "mental hygiene." The concept of the self, along with the pragmatism of James that influenced George Herbert Mead to help pioneer sociology in America resulting in the posthumously published Mind, Self, and Society (1934). Research in the sociology of mental health not only shares this history with psychology and medicine, but also the very foundation of sociology in America. The earliest sociological research in Europe, from Durkheim's study of suicide to Simmel's most famous mental life in the metropolis, manifested an unmistakable concern with the mental health of its subjects. This common core is rarely noted within most sociological perspectives that appear to view mental health research as distant or distinct from the central tenets of our discipline, or worse yet, owing allegiance or deference to the interests and corrupting influences of the more powerful disciplines noted above. The impact of research in the sociology of mental health makes clear that neither could be farther from the truth. The foundations and interests are more accurately portrayed as common, with the impact and influence of research on the sociology of mental health deriving substantially from contributions to sociological perspectives.

These successes were evident throughout the middle years of the last (twentieth) century and became a prominent feature in the landscape of sociological research by the last third of that century. Some of these early foundations and their continuing influence throughout the twentieth century can be traced in several of the chapters in this monograph. By way of a few examples, Carpiano provides insights from the "past as prologue to the present," Watson, McCranie and Wright sketch out a "cultural history of recovery," and Link and Phelan trace the development of the concept of stigma from the 1950s and 1960s till today. A detailed and comprehensive history of the sociology of mental health research has yet to be produced and is beyond the scope of a monograph such as this one, but these examples and others found in the chapters of this monograph provide a notion of how productive and useful the exploration of this topic would be. In the end, however, the monograph format required us to select just a few topics to illustrate their place in the legacy of mental health research in sociology. And just as a lengthier and more comprehensive history could be written for each one of them, a broader and more comprehensive list of topics would have to be covered in order to provide the complete legacy of that research, which this monograph only begins to address.

Topics Covered

The manuscripts in this monograph provide us with some thoughts about where the sociology of mental health research has led us, and where it is going. This is only a sampling of the important topics in the field, by no means all, but each is a fitting contribution to the commemoration of the field as a whole and especially of the specific topic. There is need for more of this work to be done on other topics in other areas, and in the opinion of more than one reviewer, these chapters provide a model for such future work. The topics include social support, stigma and labeling, gender and marital status, the stress process, mental health care, the effects of neighborhoods, and an assessment of the legacy of mental health research in sociology.

Social Support

Social relationships are a fundamental cause, in a salutatory sense as thoroughly documented and well explained by Turner, Turner and Hale., but they can also be pathogenic in terms of trauma inflicted, emotional pain evoked, and even disease transmitted (common cold)/infected(HIV)/inflicted or spread (biological warfare), toxins and carcinogens exposed, etc. Social relationships sooth and wound, heal and kill. Understanding these social relationships are not only fundamental to explaining the cause of health and illness, but also the fundamental concepts that help us understand the science of sociology itself. One can hardly imagine a concept more important to the sociology of mental health researchers, let alone sociologists in general.

Turner, Turner and Hale locate the roots of modern day interest in social support in the seminal ideas and concepts of Cassel and Cobb. The authors follow this exposition by introducing the reader to the massive accomplishments that have occurred since those early statements pointing out that many of the achievements were contributions from members of section on the sociology of mental health. Readers are introduced to the accumulated evidence concerning whether and to what extent social support has main effects, buffering effects, or both in relation to stressful circumstances. Evidence is also provided concerning the challenge of selection effects in relation to associations between perceived support and health, the role of support in accounting for gender, SES, and other health disparities. The chapter also considers the important possibility that not all social embeddedness is beneficial to health and ends with an account of the major things we have learned about support as it relates to mental and physical health.

Stigma and Labeling

Beginning with the foundation of stigma laid by Goffman (1963) in the early 1960s and building at first on its link to labeling theory, Link and Phelan show how these important sociological concepts play a fundamental role in the sociological understanding of the persistence and consequences of mental illness. The chapter describes theoretical advances, reviews studies of public conceptions of mental illnesses, and covers research relating to the ways in which, and the extent to which, people are affected by stigma. Also provided is an effective primer on revised labeling theory and on the contributions this work is making to the sociology of mental health and to sociology more generally.

Gender and Marital Status

We are also very pleased to include gender, marital status, and emotional well-being by Simon. This chapter surveys important trends in research concerning the mental health consequences of gender and marital status. As noted by reviewers, "is a model for what a chapter of this kind should do" and "this chapter is excellent, well written and comprehensive." It is a comprehensive review of the literature that organizes it into a few general ideas, making both readily accessible to those wishing to enter into this line of research. It also is very contemporary, poses some questions that have yet to be asked or even to have occurred to many already familiar with the topics here. Simon presents the three main hypotheses about the gender disparity in mental health, differential (a) exposure to stress, (b) vulnerability and (c) gendered responses. In addition, she merges this focus on gender with the substantial literature on marital status in an attempt to explain how marriage confers mental health advantages, and speculates forward on the timely question of whether the same advantages of heterosexual marriage will apply to persons entering same-sex marriages today.

Stress Process

It has been widely noted that stress theory and the stress process model represents the dominant theory guiding sociological research on mental health and mental illness. That stress research is to be found at the very core of the sociology of mental health research is effectively demonstrated by Aneshensel and Mitchel who provide a thoughtful review of the current status of relevant theory and research. This review attends to Pearlin's contention that social stress, as well as coping resources, arise out of the context of people's lives. The evidence cited confirms the significance of each element of the stress process model, effectively linking these elements to occupancy of social statuses and roles. Importantly, as one reviewer stated, the chapter also makes a major contribution by posing "unanswered questions," not the least of which involves the "consideration of the work that remains to be done in evaluating the explanatory significance of the stress process model."

Mental Health Care

Sociology has and continues to make important contributions to our understanding of the mental health significance of social relationships. Among relationships that may be of crucial significance is that between patients and the clinical health professionals that provide assistance and care. The chapter by Watson, McCranie and Wright stakes a solid claim for the contributions sociology has made toward understanding factors that promote recovery from serious mental illness (SMI). The authors consider a topic that is documented to have a long history of inquiry, yet is notable by its relative neglect over recent years. As noted by a reviewer, it is "an important topic, and it should be in a volume focusing on the sociology of mental health. The present chapter does a good job of covering important aspects of this process." These authors describe and explain the role of a once major paradigmatic player in understanding of the sociology of mental health and illness, the social constructionist perspective. They place the topic firmly within another major area of mental health research—the use and financing of health care services, types of treatment offered and received, and their outcomes.

The Neighborhood and Mental Life

We could not agree more with one reviewer who stated that this "chapter covers one of the most important areas that have become prominent in the sociology of mental health over the past 20 years." The chapter by Carpiano likely borrows its title directly from the foundational work by Simmel as part of its nod to the past, and provides one of the better transitions covering the period from then (e.g., work done by Faris and Dunham) to modern mental health research that began in the boom era described earlier. But also, in Part II it looks to the future and will be very useful for those working or wishing to begin working in this area.

We could not agree more with one reviewer who stated that this "chapter covers one of the most important areas that have become prominent in the sociology of mental health over the past 20 years." The chapter by Carpiano situates the contributions of modern-day researchers in the context of the rich history that preceded those contributions. As part of its nod to the past, Carpaino provides a title for his chapter that follows on Simmel's class essay, "The Metropolis and Mental Life." He points to the seminal contributions of classic theory including Durkheim, Engels, and Simmel, following that exposition with a thoughtful identification of threads through the Chicago School (Faris and Dunham) and the critically important Stirling County Study (Leighton, Dohrenewend). Recent work has followed on this impressive legacy developing and extending understanding about the role of neighborhood. The reader learns from this review just how deeply the case has been made for the importance placed in the sociology of mental health. Carpiano also moves on from what the past has provided to imagine the kinds of contributions that still need to be made. One suggestion is to carefully attend specifically "for whom" a particular neighborhood effect is likely to matter and "for what" particular outcome. He then advises that major contributions still need to be made in (1) the area of neighborhood organizations and the services they provide, (2) cultural circumstances in neighborhood contexts, and (3) the critical issues of agency and health behavior. The overall conclusion is unmistakable—the study of neighborhood contexts as they pertain to mental health has a rich history and a promising future.

Legacy of Mental Health Research

This chapter is an impenitent heralding of the enormous scientific contribution, status enhancement, and public health benefits of the sociology of mental health to the public welfare and prestige of the discipline. It follows an earlier study (Johnson and Wolinsky 1990) completed just before the formation of the Section on the Sociology of Mental Health that attributed the rise in the stature of the *Journal of Health and Social Behavior* in part to the impact of stress research, which Mechanic (1990) properly pointed out was a legacy that could just as easily be attributed to mental health research as a whole given the broad operationalization of stress research in the original article. The overall conclusions from the earlier study are confirmed in this chapter, further validating the point that mental health research plays an important role in sociology in general with a notable impact within the discipline as well as across disciplines.

Topics Not Covered

The decision to offer a brief monograph in recognition of the 30th anniversary of the formation of the Section on the Sociology of Mental Health had one inescapable dysfunction: there is a vast array of research topics with a range of scientific impact that is not included. Some of these were not included because the initial survey of the impact of the field did not uncover enough evidence of the topic to reveal its potential (either emerging topics or long neglected ones). Others that were uncovered were left out simply because to include them all would turn a brief monograph into a handbook (not compatible with the form or the intent of the genre selected). There is thus a need to realize that this monograph cannot alone serve the function of fully commemorating the impact of the research in the field, and to the extent that does accomplish some of that task it should also serve as a call to expand this beyond what is covered here. We would like to suggest, in our view, what efforts are needed extend beyond the content of this commemorative monograph to other topics in mental health research. In part, this reflects both topics that have been noted to have impact in the past and well as emerging topics. They include family and work, inequality, public policy, a detailed history and foundation, the social construction and epidemiology of specific illnesses, such as depression, posttraumatic stress disorder (PTSD), anxiety, attention deficit hyperactivity disorder (ADHD), and autism spectrum disorders (to name only some). To assist in these ongoing efforts we need to understand and explore the measurement, methods, and scales used in mental health research. And there continues to be a debt owed and efforts devoted to understanding the major events of our lives and how they influence our mental health.

References

Goffman, E. (1963). *Stigma: Notes on the Management of a Spoiled Identity*. New York: Simon and Schuster.
James, W. (1890). The Hidden Self. *Scribner's Magazine, 7*(3), 361–374.
Johnson, R. J., & Wolinsky, F. D. (1990). The Legacy of Stress Research: Course and Impact of this Journal. *Journal of Health and Social Behavior, 31*(3), 217–225.
Mead, G. H. (1934). *Mind, Self and Society*. Chicago: University of Chicago Press.
Mechanic, D. (1990). Comment: The Legacy of Stress Research. *Journal of Health and Social Behavior, 31*(3), 226–227.
Simmel, G. (1903). The Metropolis and Mental Life. In K. Wolf (Ed.), 1950, *The Sociology of Georg Simmel* (pp. 409–426). Glencoe, Illinois: The Free Press.

Chapter 1
Social Relationships and Social Support

R. Jay Turner, J. Blake Turner and William Beardall Hale

As has been frequently noted, the sociology of mental health as a field of study appears to have been initially motivated by observations that mental illnesses and psychological distress are differentially distributed in the population. Numerous studies on the occurrence and prevalence of mental health problems, and on virtually all somatic diseases that have been examined, have shown reliable associations with such factors as low socioeconomic position, gender and marital status. The increasingly documented generality of these relationships across acute and chronic diseases and disorders alike argues strongly that the causal factors involved must also be quite general in nature.

Nearly four decades ago Cassel (1974, 1976) described this generality in terms of a complete absence of etiologic specificity. He argued that the social environment must function to enhance or lower susceptibility to all forms of illness in general, with the type of disorder that eventuates being determined on other grounds. At about the same time, Syme and Berkman (1976) published their interpretation of the pervasiveness of the social class-illness relationship as indicating class differences in general vulnerability. Despite a massive amount of subsequent evidence supporting these claims, most subsequent sociological research on health has focused on factors associated with specific individual disorders.

As Link and Phelan (1995: 88) have noted, "Since only one manifestation of the social cause is measured in such studies, the full impact of the social cause

---

R.J. Turner (✉) · W.B. Hale
Vanderbilt University, Nashville, USA
e-mail: r.jay.turner@vanderbilt.edu

W.B. Hale
e-mail: William.b.hale@vanderbilt.edu

J.B. Turner
Columbia University, New York, USA
e-mail: turnerb@nyspi.columbia.edu

goes unrecorded." Their now classic work on "Social Conditions as Fundamental Causes of Disease" (Link and Phelan 1995) along with the persuasive admonitions of Aneshensel (1992, 2005), Aneshensel et al. (1991) serve as reminders that the factors underlying the generality of observed social status-health linkages must also be quite general in nature.

The present chapter is centrally informed by the assumption that the social environment matters for health because it influences one's general vulnerability. Our focus is on the hypothesis that social support and social connectedness represent core determinants of such general vulnerability.

To summarize, the role and significance of social support and social connectedness are here considered from a perspective composed of three assumptions: (1) social factors must act to raise or lower risk for all forms of disease and disorder; (2) the generality of observed connections between social statuses and health suggest the likelihood that the influential mechanisms involved must also be quite general in nature; and (3) there are good grounds for proposing that social support/social connectedness represents such a general and influential factor.

The ancestry of social support research is often traced to Durkheim's ([1897] 1951) treatise and empirical assessment of the role of social involvement in the prevention of suicide. However, the well-documented boom in social support research (e.g. House et al. 1988b; Vaux 1988; Veil and Baumann 1992) followed, and was importantly stimulated by, the publication of seminal articles by Cassel (1976) and Cobb (1976). These papers introduced a hypothesis and assembled preliminary supporting evidence that the availability and quality of social relationships may act to buffer the impact of exposure to life stress. In other words, the impact of stress may be greater among those who lack social ties compared to those who have supportive relationships with others. It should be noted, however, that the health benefits of social support have also often been considered in terms of its direct and mediating effects as well as in terms of its targeted role in reducing the noxious effects of life stress (Thoits 2011).

1.1 Concepts of Social Support

"Social support" has diverse meanings. It has been variously described in such terms as social bonds, social networks, meaningful social contact, availability of confidants, and human companionship as well as social support (Turner 1983). Although these concepts are hardly identical, all are reasonably captured by one or more aspects of dictionary definitions that define support as to "keep from failing or giving way, give courage, confidence, or power of endurance to...supply with necessities.... Lend assistance or countenance to" (Oxford dictionary 1975: 850). Commensurately, *social support* involves the transference of these benefits through the presence and content of human relationships. Most conceptualizations share this clear focus on the relevance of human relationships for health—the significance of which seems difficult to overstate given accumulating evidence partially reviewed below.

Cobb (1976: 300), who provided perhaps the best known and most influential conceptualization of social support, viewed social support as comprised of information. Specifically, "information belonging to one or more of the following three classes: (1) information leading the subject to believe that he[/she] is cared for and loved; (2) information leading the subject to believe that he[/she] is esteemed and valued; and (3) information leading the subject to believe that he[/she] belongs to a network of communication and mutual obligation." In other words, perceived social support refers to the clarity or certainty with which the individual experiences being loved, valued, and able to count on others should the need arise (Lakey and Scoboria 2005).

Perceived social support has been the most prominent conceptualization in social support research since its early beginnings. This focus is consistent with W.I. Thomas's familiar admonition that situations that are defined as real are real in their consequences (Thomas and Thomas 1928). This classic perspective seems fully isomorphic with a core axiom of modern day social psychology that events and circumstances in the real world affect the individual only to the extent and in the form in which they are perceived. As Ausubel (1958: 277) long ago pointed out, "this does not imply that the perceived world is the real world but that perceptual reality is psychological reality and the actual (mediating) variable that influences behavior and development."

Empirical support for the importance of perceived support followed. In an early comprehensive review of the social support literature, House (1981) noted that the bulk of evidence for the health benefits of social support came from studies focused on "emotional support"—his term for perceived support. He further acknowledged that emotional support was the common element across most conceptualizations, that it captured what most people meant when they spoke of someone being supportive and that, indeed, it seemed to be the most important dimension. Wethington and Kessler (1986: 85) went further, documenting not only that "perceptions of support availability are more important than actual support transactions but that the latter promotes psychological adjustment through the former, as much as by practical resolutions of situational demands."

1.2 Social Support and Health

An ever-growing number of volumes and reviews document the apparent significance of perceived social support for emotional health and well-being (e.g., Brewin et al. 2000; Cohen and Syme 1985; Cohen and Willis 1985; Dean and Lin 1977; Gottlieb 1981; Kawachi and Berkman 2001; Kessler et al. 1985; Lakey and Cronin 2008; Lincoln 2000; Lincoln et al. 2005; Sarason and Sarason 1985; Sarason et al. 1990; Stice 2002; Turner 1983; Turner et al. 1983; Vaux 1988; Veil and Baumann 1992). Perhaps the largest portion of this substantial effort has addressed the hypothesis that low levels of social support increase risk for depression. Taking note of this hypothesis, Henderson (1992) identified and evaluated 35 separate studies that assessed this relationship. These studies used measures of depression that varied from brief self-report inventories to standardized interviews based on accepted diagnostic criteria. Similarly, procedures for indexing social support differed widely, varying from a single item on the presence or absence of a confidant to sophisticated multi-item interviews or questionnaires. Despite such variable assessments of both social support and depression, Henderson observed remarkable consistency across studies. Virtually all reported a clear inverse association between social support and depression, with studies employing more brief measures of one or both variable demonstrating just as strong relationships as studies employing more elaborate methods. The conclusion seems well warranted that there is a robust and reliable relationship between social support and mental health status generally, and depression in particular.

A comparable literature is also now available attesting to the direct and stress moderating significance of social support in relation to physical health. Indeed, based on a careful review of prospective mortality studies, that included consideration of various alternative hypotheses, House et al. (1988a: 544) have concluded that "Social relationships have a predictive, arguably causal, association with health in their own right."

There is also specific and consistent evidence that lack of social support is a risk factor for coronary heart disease (CHD) onset and prognosis (Bunker et al. 2003), and is associated with reduced immunological function (Uchino et al. 1996; Cohen et al. 1997) In addition, findings have been reported suggesting that social support demonstrates a main effect with respect to blood pressure (Strogatz et al. 1997) and also buffers the impact of high stress on systolic blood pressure (Karlin et al. 2003; Berkman et al. 1993). These findings are consistent with the argument Rowe and Kahn (1987) proffered more than a quarter century ago that lack of social support may be associated with greater biological aging, and hence with increased susceptibility to the diseases of aging. Finally, social support, primarily in the form of supportive or positive family relations, has been shown by a number of investigators to be of significance for substance abuse and other problem behaviors (e.g. Jessor et al. 1995; Resnick et al. 1997; Wills et al. 1997).

This mass of evidence documenting the health significance of social support notwithstanding, it is clear that not all relationships, even those that are very close, are uniformly positive (e.g. Rook 2003; Robles and Kiecolt-Glaser 2003) and that negative aspects of relationships may be even more consequential than positive aspects, at least with respect to mental health outcomes (Finch et al. 1999; Rook 1984; Newsom et al. 2005). Evidence on adverse consequences of social relationships is considered below.

1.3 Main Versus Stress-Buffering Effects of Social Support

A substantial portion of the research on the mental health effects of social support has been associated with the hypothesis—strongly articulated in the influential papers by Cassel (1976) and Cobb (1976)—that social support acts to *buffer* the effects of life stress. As Cobb (1976) argued, social support facilitates coping with crises and adaptation to change. From this perspective, there will always be some main effects simply because life is full of changes and crises, but it is in moderating the effects of the major transitions in life and of the unexpected crises that the major effects of social support should be found.

Henderson's (1992) review of 35 social support-depression studies revealed only four that did not report this kind of buffering or protective effect. However, it is also clear from Henderson's review, and from the wider literature, that a number of studies have found a low level of support to increase risk for depression, or for mental health problems generally, whether or not exposure to unusual stressors has also taken place. A more recent review concludes that the stress-buffering effects of social support are "less dramatic and consistent" than the direct effects of social support on mental health (Thoits 2011: 145). Whether these findings allow the conclusion that social support can be of importance in the absence of social stress cannot be easily answered. Antonovsky (1979: 77) long ago argued that "all of us… even in the most benign and sheltered environments, are fairly continuously exposed to what we define as stressors…. We are able to get low scores on stress experience [only] because we do not ask the right questions or do not ask patiently enough and not because there really are any low scorers." He insists that "even the most fortunate of people…know life as stressful to a considerable extent" (1979: 79). If this constancy-of-stress argument is accepted, both the main effects and interactive effects that have been observed would theoretically be interpretable in terms of the buffering hypothesis.

Commenting on the main effects versus buffering question, Berkman and Glass (2000) have suggested that different components of social support may exert different influences on mental health. Specifically, it may be that structural and objective aspects of social relationships, such as the number of friends an individual has or the frequency of contact with these friends, yield main effects. In contrast, they hypothesize that perceived social support is likely to operate through a stress-buffering mechanism. Thoits (2011) suggests that, while the general health benefits of social support may operate through many mechanisms, the effectiveness of the support as a stress-buffer requires actually received or enacted support and is based on very specific combinations of *type* of support and *source* of support. Specifically, *love, caring, sympathy and instrumental assistance* are hypothesized to be the most effective stress-buffers when coming from *significant others*, while *validation of feelings, advice, and role modeling* are most helpful coming from *similar others*—that is, those who have experienced or are experiencing a similar stressor.

At this point, available evidence continues to suggest that social support matters for mental health independent of stressor level. Although less consistently demonstrated in the literature, most research also suggests that support matters more under circumstances of elevated stress exposure.

1.4 The Causation-Selection Debate

Research on the social correlates of health is typically conducted with the expectation that there is an etiological message to be found within well demonstrated linkages. However, in the case of social support, as with other social variables, it has been difficult to reach a clear conclusion about the nature of this message. Most of the studies reporting this relationship have been cross sectional in nature and thus have confronted the classic interpretive problem. Does perceived social support operate directly or indirectly to make depression or psychological distress less likely or less severe (social causation), or do high levels of distress or depression limit the likelihood that the individual will secure and maintain social relationships or experience the social support that is available (social selection)?

With respect to these particular alternatives, it now seems generally accepted that variations in risk for mental health problems are, to a substantial degree, socially influenced and are not wholly or even largely reducible to psychology or biology. There seem good grounds for the claim that stress research and the stress process model (Pearlin 1989; Pearlin et al. 1981; Avison et al. 2010), more than any other tradition, has demonstrated that inequalities in mental health arise out of social experiences that are importantly conditioned by the context within which lives are led (Pearlin 1989). Specifically, longitudinal studies in which prior symptoms or disorder are controlled have made it highly unlikely that the social support—distress relationship wholly or even largely reflects reverse causation (Aneshensel and Frerichs 1982; Coyne and Downey 1991; Kessler et al. 1985; Myers et al. 1972; Pearlin et al. 1981; Thoits 1995; Turner and Noh 1988).

A second form of social selection proposes that the observed social support-mental health connection may simply be an artifact derived from the personal inadequacies of persons who later become distressed or depressed—inadequacies that also limit one's ability to secure and maintain supportive relationships. That is, it is dispositional characteristics, as opposed to the nature of the social environment, that largely account for differences in perceived social support—characteristics that are also associated with increased risk for mental health problems.

In support of this contention, there is some evidence that perceived social support is fairly stable over time and associated more with personality characteristics than with variation in social interaction. Goodwin et al. (2004) found perceived social support to be more strongly related to stably held personal values than to social support actually received. Similarly, Cukrowicz et al. (2008) reported a strong correlation between personality characteristics that are negatively associated with depression and perceived social support. These findings are consistent with older research that demonstrated temporal and cross situational consistency in perceived social support (Sarason et al. 1990), and associations of these perceptions with personality characteristics such as social competence and personal control (e.g. Lakey and Cassady 1990).

Thus, at least part of the association between social support and mental health may be due to a linkage between personality characteristics and measures of both perceptions of social support and mental health. The question of how much of this association can be attributed to personality differences has been recently estimated by Turner et al. (2012) based on a large scale community based study (n = 1,859). Following Turner et al. (2004) they considered the personal attributes of mastery (Pearlin and Schooler 1978), self-esteem (Rosenberg 1979), mattering (Rosenberg and McCullough 1981), and emotional reliance (Hirschfeld et al. 1977). Having confirmed within cross sectional analyses that each of the four resources or attributes significantly and independently predict depressive symptoms, perceived social support assessed 3 years later was regressed on these attributes with demographics held constant.

With the exception of emotional reliance, all four resources were significantly associated with subsequent perceptions of social support when considered separately, with just mattering independently predicting higher support when considered together. Collectively, the personal attributes considered accounted for 5.2 % of observed variation in subsequent perceptions of social support availability.

These findings are supportive of the contention that the tendency to believe or perceive others to be supportive is at least partially a reflection of relatively stable personal attributes (Sarason et al. 1990; Lakey and Cassady 1990). As Lakey and Dickinson (1994) have suggested, higher levels of these personal resources may well signal greater effectiveness in developing and maintaining supportive relationships and a tendency to interpret ambiguous actions and statements as supportive in nature.

Thus, these results might be seen as consistent with the contention that the apparent linkage between perceived social support and mental health may be partially, if not largely, artifactual in nature. However, the strength of the associations observed suggest that personal attributes condition perceived social support to only a very modest extent. In our view, these results do not materially challenge the view that the perceived availability of social support is largely a function of one's history of supportive and unsupportive experiences (Turner and Turner 1999) and that the persistently observed linkage between social support and mental health has both theoretical and practical meaning.

1.5 Social Status and Social Support

Thus, it follows that variations in the availability and experience of social support arise primarily out of life conditions, current and past (Pearlin 1989). To the extent that important differences in such conditions are defined by incumbency in a particular set of social groups and statuses, the hypothesis follows that observed relationships between these statuses and mental health may arise, at least in part, from associated differences in social support. We therefore review evidence describing how social support may link multiple core social statuses to mental health, including socioeconomic status (SES), race/ethnicity, and gender. Marital status is excluded from this effort based on the judgment that most available evidence on the association between marital status and social support may be of only historical interest. The dramatic transformation in marital patterns and living situations over the past dozen or so years requires a reexamination of the formal relational circumstances under which the experience of being supported by others is maximized and minimized.

1.5.1 Gender

Although a substantial number of studies have provided social support data by gender, the question of sex differences in level of support experienced remains a matter of some debate. More than two decades ago, Vaux (1988: 169) accomplished a rather complete review of available evidence and concluded that "empirical findings regarding gender differences in social support are mixed and inconsistent." However, others read essentially the same evidence as indicating a tendency for women to experience more supportive relationships than men (Flaherty and Richman 1986; Leavy 1983). More recently, analyzing data from a national probability sample, Umberson et al. (1996) found clear and dramatic gender differences in the number and quality of social relationships. Women reported greater formal and informal social integration and more support from their friends. In terms of familial support, women reported more support from their adult children while married men reported greater support from their spouses than married women. In general, the weight of the evidence appears to suggest that women are advantaged with respect to social support, variously conceived and measured (Matthews et al. 1999; Ross and Mirowsky 1989; Turner and Marino 1994).

Confidence in this conclusion is bolstered by substantial evidence of gender differences in the propensity to affiliate with others. Joiner (2011) has presented compelling analyses demonstrating that men, compared to women, are much less likely to maintain and/or replace personal and social relationships across the life course. His research reveals that a crucial consequence of this failure is a largely unacknowledged loneliness that dramatically increases risk for suicide and for premature death from other causes. Evidence has long been available indicating that, in stressful circumstances, women are more likely to provide support, and to both seek and secure support, primarily from other women (Belle 1987; Luckow et al. 1998; Schachter 1959). As Taylor et al. (2000: 418) have noted, "Adult women maintain more same-sex close relationships than do men, they mobilize more social support in times of stress than do men, they rely less heavily than do men on their spouses for social support, they turn to female friends more often, they report more benefits from contact with their female friends and relatives…and they provide more frequent and more effective social support to others than do men." There are likely a number of reasons for gender differences in the propensity to affiliate with others, including cultural and role prescriptions, as well as evolved biobehavioral responses (e.g., Taylor et al. 2000), but the overall evidence for greater social connectedness among women, particularly in times of stress, is clear.

While women experience higher levels of social support than men, there appears to be little in the way of gender differences in the strength of the association between social support and mental health (e.g. Umberson et al. 1996). Thus, social support differences cannot, in any straightforward way, assist our understanding of the tendency for women to experience higher levels of psychological distress and depression. Indeed, without the advantage of higher social support, women "would exhibit even higher levels of depression relative to men than they currently do (Umberson et al. 1996, p.854)." This may be in part because the larger social networks of women render them more exposed to the adversities experienced by others (Kessler and McLeod 1984; Turner and Avison 1989). Furthermore, women are more likely than men to report becoming involved when network members experience a negative event (Wethington et al. 1987). Thus, when all aspects of social relationships are considered—the negative aspects as well as the supportive ones—the mental health advantage for women is likely to be attenuated.

1.5.2 Socioeconomic Status

To the extent that the structures and processes of social relationships vary in a systematic fashion across socioeconomic statuses, this variation may play a role in SES gradients in mental health. Here, as with the other social statuses considered, evidence bearing on this possibility, is sparse and variable. For example, the SES-social support relationship appears to vary depending on the source of support considered. Studies of adolescents and young adults indicate that SES is related to social support from family but not to support from friends (Gayman et al. 2010; Salonna et al. 2012; However, also see Huurre et al. 2007).

The operational definition of SES also can affect the results. While Ross and Mirowsky (1989) observed a positive association between education and social support, they also found that support and family income were entirely unrelated. More recently, Mickelson and Kubzansky (2003) found that education and income were independently and positively related to emotional support when different sources of support were combined, though the effects of income were observed primarily in terms of substantially diminished levels of support at the lowest levels. Research on education and social capital points to the possibility that education benefits support due in part to an enhancement of social language, and communication skills that are useful in social interactions (Glaeser et al. 2002).

Finally, the association of SES and social support is sometimes contingent on the group under study. For example, Beatty et al. (2011) assessed the developmental importance of childhood SES on adult experiences of social support. They found that supportive interactions, reported in real-time using electronic diaries, were positively associated with childhood SES, as were global perceptions of social support and reports of general network involvement. These associations remained when adult SES was controlled. They were observed, however, only for African-Americans; no effect of childhood SES among Whites was found.

Though the relationship of social support to SES is quite consistent in the literature, the extent to which support explains the SES gradient in well-being is less clear. For example, Turner and Marino (1994) indicated that social support differences explained only about 15 % of SES differences in depressive symptoms and virtually none of the observed SES variations in depressive disorders. Similar results were found for depressive symptoms more recently by Huurre et al. (2007). Thus, although childhood and adult SES appear to be important predictors of social support, the extent to which the accumulation of these resources explains SES differences in mental health is limited.

1.5.3 Race/Ethnicity

In terms of the distribution of social support across social statuses, race and ethnic groups have been comparatively understudied. Some evidence suggests that racial and ethnic minorities rely on informal sources of support, primarily family members, because of social barriers to access to other advantageous social connections (Landale et al. 2006). This tendency has been ascribed, in particular, to Latinos in the U.S. and the term *familism* has been applied to the close ties among members of large kin networks in the Latino community (Vega and Miranda 1985).

Using data from a large probability sample of Chicago residents, Almeida et al. (2009) examined the distribution of levels of perceived social support across race/ethnicity, nativity, and socioeconomic status. Latinos, and in particular Mexican-Americans, reported the highest levels of familial social support. Non-Latino Whites reported the lowest levels, with Blacks in the middle. Interestingly, the Latino advantage was attenuated with distance from circumstances characteristic of initial immigration. Specifically, the advantage largely disappeared among Latinos living in English-speaking households and the SES-familial social support gradient among Latinos was negative. That is, familial support decreased with increasing SES—a finding opposite to that observed for Blacks and non-Latino Whites. These findings are consistent with the familism hypothesis.

In contrast to familial social support, Latinos reported the lowest levels of friend support. Non-Latino whites reported the highest levels with Blacks again in the middle. A strong positive SES gradient with friend support existed across the race/ethnic groups, indicating that access to non-familial supportive networks is another resource accruing differentially to the socially advantaged (Almeida et al. 2009).

Some apparent race/ethnic differences in social support could actually be measurement artifacts. If questions asked about social support are interpreted differently across groups, or if there are cultural differences in the tendencies to endorse a social support item at similar levels of actual support, then biased estimates of race/ethnic differences could result. Sacco et al. (2011) assessed differential item functioning (DIF) across five race/ethnic groups in the US. DIF assesses differences across groups in the propensity to endorse particular items at the same levels of the underlying latent construct—in this case, social support. These researchers found DIF for every item in their perceived support measure, with Blacks and Hispanics responding differently from whites. However, it is important to note that these groups showed lower levels support relative to whites on the unadjusted measure, a finding opposite to those cited above. Thus, it appears that the presence of DIF across race/ethnic groups is, itself, likely to be very different depending on the social support measure used.

Overall, this research suggests that race and ethnicity are important factors in the distribution of social support, particularly in intersection with SES. Differences in social support across these groups are important considerations in the study of the epidemiology of mental health. Researchers should be mindful of the potential for cultural differences in response tendencies to questions about social support. Finally, more research examining the role of social support in race and ethnic differences in mental health is needed.

1.6 Further Considerations

1.6.1 Social Integration Versus Relationship Content

In a critical review of the social support literature published more than two decades ago, House et al. (1988a) emphasized the importance of assessing social integration (the existence and structure of social relationships) independent of relationship content (quality and valence of the relationships, reliability of support, etc.). Separate assessment of these two constructs facilitates an examination of the processes through which social relationships translate into the experience of social support, and the structural factors that influence these processes. They argue that the reviewed evidence supports the proposition that the presence of social relationships have important effects on health and well-being separately from, and irrespective of, the content of those relationships.

Recent findings on the issue are mixed. Analyzing data from large epidemiological surveys in the U.S. and Taiwan, Son et al. (2008) found that levels of social integration had substantially weaker associations with depression than did the presence of a close confidant. Falci and McNeely (2009), in contrast, found that network size was importantly related to depressive symptoms in adolescents independent of the presence of a confident. Interestingly, the relationship was not linear—social networks that were unusually large and unusually small were both related to elevated symptoms. Low perceptions of friend support partially explained the adverse effects of small networks but not of unusually large networks.

If the mere presence of social relationships enhances health and emotional well-being, irrespective of the supportive content of the relationships, then mechanisms for such an effect need to be considered and examined—mechanisms that do not involve cognitive appraisal or behavioral coping. For physical health, Umberson (1987) has suggested that social networks act to facilitate health-promoting behaviors (diet, exercise, etc.) through the instrumental assistance they provide and restrict noxious behaviors (smoking, drinking, etc.). Antonovsky (1979) has suggested a more general mechanism in which social integration is an important contributor to an individual's "sense of coherence." Sense of coherence, in Antonovsky's view, diminishes reactivity to stress and is an important component of psychological well-being in its own right. Finally, the direct neuroendocrine sequelae of contact with other human beings and the health consequences of these reactions is a growing area of investigation and one that clearly deserves attention (Kiecolt-Glaser et al. 2010).

1.6.2 Negative Aspects of Social Relationships

Researchers in the area of the sociology of mental health, particularly those working within the stress process paradigm, have generally considered the negative aspects of social relationships to be a component of stress exposure (Pearlin et al. 1981). In this conceptualization, exposure to social negativity—criticisms and/or unreasonable expectations from socially significant others—is potentially moderated by social support and other personal resources (Thoits 2011). However, if we view social support as a factor on which we hope to intervene to improve population mental health, then it is important to be mindful of the potential adverse effects of social interactions.

The available evidence suggests that such adverse effects can be substantial (Lincoln 2000; Turner 1994). This may be especially true with respect to what Rook (2001) and others have referred to as negative social exchanges. Examples of such exchanges include "discouraging the expression of feelings, making critical remarks, invading another's privacy…(and) failing to provide promised help" (Lincoln 2000: 233). Not only does a significant amount of the extant literature suggest harmful effects from such negative exchanges (e.g., Finch et al. 1989; Lakey et al. 1994; Revenson et al. 1991; Ruehlman and Karoly 1991; Pagel et al. 1987), it suggests that these effects may be greater than the benefits to mental health provided by the social relationships (e.g., Lincoln 2000; Horwitz et al. 1998; Reinhardt 2001). Examining data from the National Comorbidity Study, Bertera (2005) found that social negativity was associated far more strongly with episodes of anxiety and mood disorders than was positive support. Given the cross sectional nature of these data and of most other studies reporting such effects, the possibility should be considered that the causation involved in observed negative interaction-distress relationships may well be more bi-directional in nature than is the case with positive interactions and perceptions, thereby inflating the magnitude of the negative interaction associations. Using data from a large survey of adults over the age of 50 in Great Britain, Stafford et al. (2011) found the adverse effects of negative social exchanges (in this case on levels of depressive symptoms) to be pervasive across social relationships. In their data, positive exchanges had beneficial effects when they involved spouses and children, but not when they came from other relatives or friends. The greater importance of negative interactions has also been reported based on a U.S. national sample of elderly African-Americans (Lincoln et al. 2010). In this study, emotional support was unrelated to the odds of a lifetime diagnosis of anxiety or depression. In contrast, negative interactions were strongly related to an increased likelihood of both disorders. However, since it is clear that disorder onsets occurred prior to the assessment of emotional support these findings may simply indicate that psychiatric disorders better predict subsequent negative interactions than they predict lower levels of perceived emotional support.

However, in their longitudinal study of older adults, Newsom et al. (2003) examined the association of positive and negative social exchanges to positive and negative affect, both cross-sectionally and longitudinally. Cross-sectionally, the associations were valence-specific—that is, negative social exchanges were associated with negative affect and positive social exchanges with positive affect. The longitudinal analysis provided a very different picture. Positive social exchanges were not related to subsequent changes in either outcome. In contrast, negative social exchanges were associated both with subsequent increases in negative affect and with subsequent reductions in positive affect.

August et al. (2007) examined the joint effects of negative social exchanges and stressful life events. Negative social exchanges were more strongly associated with emotional distress when they occurred in the context of a major stressful experience. The interesting exception was relationship loss. Negative social interaction actually showed reduced effects on emotional distress in the context of a relationship loss, a finding the investigators surmise was due to the reduced salience of negative interaction in the context of such a loss, or to a greater appreciation for remaining relationships that makes negative interactions less stressful.

Clearly more research capable of establishing time ordering and effectively ruling out major competing explanations is needed. However, from present knowledge, it seems clear that any attempt to understand the stress-buffering effects of social relationships, as opposed to perceived social support, will obtain misleading results if the adverse aspects of relationships are not considered in tandem.

1.6.3 Interventions and Levels of Analysis

Part of the attractiveness of social support to social researchers presumably derives from the view that it is amenable to intervention. Indeed, the dominant research question of the social support field, buffering versus main effects, has been motivated partly by the goal of identifying appropriate intervention targets based on need. But is the idea of targeted intervention the most useful one? Even if the preponderance of the individual-level influence of social support is due to stress buffering, the largest public mental health effects may be more likely to result from macrolevel changes addressed to the social integration of communities. By definition, macrolevel changes are, in Ryan's (1971) terminology, "universalistic" rather than "exceptionalistic". Exceptionalistic interventions can only benefit those who are specifically targeted. In contrast, the influence of macro-level dimensions of social contact (social integration, community-level social cohesion, and connectedness) on health and well-being tends to be discernible largely or wholly at an aggregate level of analysis. For example, commenting on the substantial differences in coronary heart disease (CHD) mortality and morbidity rates between Framingham, Massachusetts, and Reno, Nevada, Lynch (1977) attributed the contrast to the fact that Reno residents were predominately recent arrivals and had few ties to the community. Framingham's population consisted primarily of lifetime residents with strong community ties. However, it does not necessarily follow, as Lynch argued, that geographically mobile, less socially connected individuals have a greater risk of CHD. It may instead be that lack of social cohesion and connectedness at the community level has noxious effects on the community as a whole irrespective of individual social circumstances. Durkheim (1951) explained and understood his findings on the correlates of suicide risk at this level of analysis.

Umberson and Montez (2010) discuss the policy implications of our knowledge regarding the health benefits of social ties. Noting that positive marital interaction fosters health and well-being for children as well as for their parents, they praise the Healthy Marriage Initiative which includes public awareness campaigns on healthy marriages and responsible parenting as well as educational and counseling services. Given that the health consequences of social isolation are well-documented and potentially severe, they advocate enhancement of the educational system so as to impart social-emotional skills and promote civic engagement. Recognizing that the burdens and negative features of social ties are not randomly distributed in the population, they argue for policies to assist caregivers. While ambitious, however, most of the policies suggested are essentially exceptionalistic, often involving identification of, and outreach to, socially isolated individuals in the community. Umberson and Montez (2010) correctly point out that very little is yet known about the ways in which the larger social context shapes social ties. Hence, social policies that might foster universalistic improvements in the quality of social life are not yet available.

It is possible, however, to examine the characteristics and social policies of societies doing very well in terms of emotional well-being. For example, large international surveys consistently place Denmark among the happiest countries in the world. That this is a country in which 92 % of the population belong to government–funded social clubs (Buettner 2010), at least suggests an avenue for a large scale policy intervention for the improvement of social ties and social integration.

1.7 Conclusions

Despite the huge body of research on social support, much remains to be learned about how and why social support matters for health and well-being, and about the circumstances and processes that promote and enhance its availability. Several conclusions, however, are warranted from available evidence.

1. The ever growing number of studies and reviews on the subject leave little doubt that social support is importantly associated with mental health status in general, and depression in particular.
2. Social support tends to matter for psychological distress and depression independent of stress level. However, it tends to matter more to both individuals and communities where stress exposure is relatively high.
3. Perceived availability of social support tends to be much more strongly related to psychological distress and depression than reports of support actually received.
4. An expanded focus on the mental health relevance of social ties and on ways to intervene to improve social support requires that we be mindful that social relationships have negative as well as positive components.
5. Levels of social support vary reliably with location in the social system as defined by SES, gender, race/ethnicity, and perhaps marital status. This suggests that the experience of being supported by others arises substantially out of social experience. Evidence indicating that social support explains status-based differences in mental health is more limited, however.

In summary, when considering the issue of social support and mental health, it is useful to acknowledge that most causes and effects in human affairs are likely to be reciprocal in nature. In the present case, evidence suggests that the perceived availability of social support has important consequences for distress and depression. At the same time, it is probable that one's mental health status and personality characteristics affect the availability of social support and the ability or tendency to experience the support that is available. Social support is important for mental health, but a variety of social and psychological conditions are important influences on social support. Additional research that clarifies the causal ordering of these relationships and their interrelated nature is critical for an understanding of the social bases of mental health.

References

Almeida, J., Johnson, R. M., Corliss, H. L., Molnar, B. E., & Azrael, D. (2009). Emotional distress among LGBT youth: The influence of perceived discrimination based on sexual orientation. *Journal of Youth and Adolescence, 38*(7), 1001–1014.

Aneshensel, C. S. (1992). Social stress: Theory and research. *Annual Review of Sociology, 18*, 15–38.

Aneshensel, C. S. (2005). Research in mental health: Social etiology versus social consequences. *Journal of Health and Social Behavior, 46*(3), 221–228.

Aneshensel, C. S., & Frerichs, R. R. (1982). Stress, support, and depression: A longitudinal causal model. *Journal of Community Psychology, 10*(4), 363–376.

Aneshensel, C. S., Rutter, C. M., & Lachenbruch, P. A. (1991). Social structure, stress, and mental health: Competing conceptual and analytic models. *American Sociological Review, 56*(2), 166–178.

Antonovsky, A. (1979). *Health, stress, and coping*. San Francisco: Jossey-Bass.

August, K. J., Rook, K. S., & Newsom, J. T. (2007). The joint effects of life stress and negative social exchanges on emotional distress. *The Journals of Gerontology Series B: Psychological Sciences and Social Sciences, 62*(5), S304–S314.

Ausubel, D. P. (1958). *Theory and problems of child development*. New York: Grune & Stratton.

Avison, W. R., Aneshensel, C. S., Schieman, S., & Wheaton, B. (2010). *Advances in the conceptualization of the stress process: Essays in honor of Leonard I.* New York: Springer.

Beatty, D. L., Kamarck, T. W., Matthews, K. A., & Shiffman, S. (2011). Childhood socioeconomic status is associated with psychosocial resources in African Americans: The Pittsburgh healthy heart project. *Health Psychology, 30*(4), 472–480.

Belle, D. (1987). Gender differences in the social moderators of stress. In R. C. Barnett, L. Biener, & G. K. Baruch (Eds.), *Gender and stress*. New York: Free Press.

Berkman, L. F., & Glass, T. A. (2000). Social integration, social networks, social support, and health. In L. F. Berkman & I. Kawachi (Eds.), *Social epidemiology* (pp. 137–173). New York: Oxford Press.

Berkman, L. F., Vaccarino, T. E., & Seeman, V. (1993). Gender differences in cardiovascular morbidity and mortality: The contribution of social networks and support. *Annals of Behavioral Medicine, 15*(2/3), 112–118.

Bertera, E. M. (2005). Mental health in U.S. adults: The role of positive social support and social negativity in personal relationships. *Journal of Social and Personal Relationships, 22*(1), 33–48.

Brewin, C. R., Andrews, B., & Valentine, J. D. (2000). Meta-analysis of risk factors for post-traumatic stress disorder in trauma-exposed adults. *Journal of Consulting and Clinical Psychology, 68*(5), 748–766.

Buettner, D. (2010). *The blue zones: Lessons for living longer from the people who've lived the longest.* Washington, DC: National Geographic.

Bunker, S. J., Colquhoun, D. M., Esler, M. D., Hickie, I. B., David Hunt, V., Jelinek, M., et al. (2003). 'Stress' and coronary heart disease: Psychosocial risk factors. *Medical Journal of Australia, 178*(6), 272–276.

Cassel, J. (1974). An epidemiological perspective of psychosocial factors in disease etiology. *American Journal of Public Health, 64*(11), 1040.

Cassel, J. (1976). The contribution of the social environment to host resistance. *American Journal of Epidemiology, 104*(2), 107–123.

Cobb, S. (1976). Presidential Address-1976. Social support as a moderator of life stress. *Psychosomatic Medicine, 38*(5), 300–314.

Cohen, S., Doyle, W. J., Skoner, D. P., Rabin, B. S., & Gwaltney, J. M, Jr. (1997). Social ties and susceptibility to the common cold. *JAMA, 277*(24), 1940–1944.

Cohen, S., & Syme, S. L. (Eds.). (1985). *Social support and health.* New York: Academic Press.

Cohen, S., & Willis, T. A. (1985). Stress, social support, and the buffering hypothesis. *Psychological Bulletin, 98*(2), 310–357.

Coulson, J. (1975). In J. Coulson, D. Eagle, J. Hawkins & H. M. Petter (Eds.), *The Oxford illustrated dictionary* (2nd ed.). Oxford: Oxford University Press.

Coyne, J. C., & Downey, G. (1991). Social factors and psychopathology: Stress, social support, and coping processes. *Annual Review of Psychology, 42*(1), 401–425.

Cukrowicz, K. C., Franzese, A. T., Thorp, S. R., Cheavens, J. S., & Lynch, T. R. (2008). Personality traits and perceived social support among depressed older adults. *Aging and Mental Health, 12,* 662–669.

Dean, A., & Lin, N. (1977). The stress-buffering role of social support: Problems and prospects for systematic investigation. *The Journal of Nervous and Mental Disease, 165*(6), 403–417.

Durkheim, É. (1951). *Suicide: A study in sociology* [1897]. New York: Simon & Schuster.

Falci, C., & McNeely, C. (2009). Too many friends: Social integration, network cohesion and adolescent depressive symptoms. *Social Forces, 87,* 2031–2061.

Finch, J. F., Okun, M. A., Barrera, M., Zautra, A. J., & Reich, J. W. (1989). Positive and negative social ties among older adults: Measurement models and the prediction of psychological distress and well-being. *American Journal of Community Psychology, 17*(5), 585–605.

Finch, J. F., Okun, M. A., Pool, G. J., & Ruehlman, L. S. (1999). A comparison of the influence of conflictual and supportive social interactions on psychological distress. *Journal of Personality, 67*(4), 581–621.

Flaherty, J. A., & Richman, J. A. (1986). Effects of childhood relationships on the adult's capacity to form social supports. *The American Journal of Psychiatry, 143*(7), 851–855.

Gayman, M. D., Turner, R. J., Cislo, A. M., & Eliassen, A. H. (2010). Early adolescent family experiences and perceived social support in young adulthood. *The Journal of Early Adolescence, 31*(6), 880–908.

Glaeser, E. L., Laibson, D., & Sacerdote, B. (2002). An economic approach to social capital. *The Economic Journal, 112*(483), F437–F458.

Goodwin, R., Costa, P., & Adonu, J. (2004). Social support and its consequences: 'Positive' and 'deficiency' values and their implications for support and self-esteem. *The British Journal of Social Psychology, 43*(Pt 3), 465–474.

Gottlieb, B. H. (1981). Social networks and social support in community mental health. In B. H. Gottlieb & B. Hills (Eds.), *Social networks and social support* (pp. 11–41). Beverley Hills, CA: Sage Publications.

Henderson, H. O. F. (1992). Social support and depression. In *The meaning and measurement of social support* (pp. 1–7). New York: Hemisphere.

Hirschfeld, R. M. A., Klerman, G. L., Gouch, H. G., Barrett, J., Korchin, S. J., & Chodoff, P. (1977). A measure of interpersonal dependency. *Journal of Personality Assessment, 41*(6), 610–618.

Horwitz, A. V., McLaughlin, J., & White, H. R. (1998). How the negative and positive aspects of partner relationships affect the mental health of young married people. *Journal of Health and Social Behavior, 39*(2), 124–136.

House, J. S. (1981). *Work stress and social support*. Reading, MA: Addison-Wesley.
House, J. S., Landis, K. R., & Umberson, D. (1988a). Social relationships and health. *Science, 241*(4865), 540–545.
House, J. S., Umberson, D., & Landis, K. R. (1988b). Structures and processes of social support. *Annual Review of Sociology, 14*, 293–318.
Huurre, T., Eerola, M., Rahkonen, O., & Aro, H. (2007). Does social support affect the relationship between socioeconomic status and depression? A longitudinal study from adolescence to adulthood. *Journal of Affective Disorders, 100*(1–3), 55–64.
Jessor, R., Van Den Bos, J., Vanderryn, J., Costa, F. M., & Turbin, M. S. (1995). Protective factors in adolescent problem behavior: Moderator effects and developmental change. *Developmental Psychology, 31*(6), 923–933.
Joiner, T. E. (2011). *Lonely at the top*. New York: MacMillan.
Karlin, W. A., Brondolo, E., & Schwartz, J. (2003). Workplace social support and ambulatory cardiovascular activity in New York City traffic agents. *Psychosomatic Medicine, 65*(2), 167–176.
Kawachi, I., & Berkman, L. F. (2001). Social ties and mental health. *Journal of Urban Health: Bulletin of the New York Academy of Medicine, 78*(3), 458–467.
Kessler, R. C., & McLeod, J. D. (1984). Sex differences in vulnerability to undesirable life events. *American Sociological Review, 49*(5), 620–631.
Kessler, R. C., Price, R. H., & Wortman, C. B. (1985). Social factors in psychopathology: Stress, social support, and coping processes. *Annual Review of Psychology, 36*(1), 531.
Kiecolt-Glaser, J. K., Gouin, J.-P., & Hantsoo, L. (2010). Close relationships, inflammation, and health. *Neuroscience and Biobehavioral Reviews, 35*(1), 33–38.
Lakey, B., & Cassady, P. B. (1990). Cognitive processes in perceived social support. *Journal of Personality and Social Psychology, 59*(2), 337–343.
Lakey, B., Cronin, A. (2008). Low social support and major depression. In *Risk factors for depression* (pp. 385–408). San Diego, CA: Academic Press.
Lakey, B., & Dickinson, L. G. (1994). Antecedents of perceived support: Is perceived family environment generalized to new social relationships? *Cognitive Therapy and Research, 18*(1), 39–53.
Lakey, B., & Scoboria, A. (2005). The relative contribution of trait and social influences to the links among perceived social support, affect, and self-esteem. *Journal of Personality, 73*(2), 361–388.
Lakey, B., Tardiff, T. A., & Drew, J. B. (1994). Negative social interactions: Assessment and relations to social support, cognition, and psychological distress. *Journal of Social and Clinical Psychology, 13*(1), 42–62.
Landale, N. S., Oropesa, R. S., & Bradatan, C. (2006). Hispanic families in the United States: Family structure and process in an era of family change. In M. Tienda & F. Mitchell (Eds.), *Hispanics and the future of America*. Washington, DC: The National Academies Press.
Leavy, R. L. (1983). Social support and psychological disorder: A review. *Journal of Community Psychology, 11*, 3–21.
Lincoln, K. D. (2000). Social support, negative social interactions, and psychological well-being. *The Social Service Review, 74*(2), 231–252.
Lincoln, K. D., Chatters, L. M., & Taylor, R. J. (2005). Social support, traumatic events, and depressive symptoms among African Americans. *Journal of Marriage and the Family, 67*(3), 754–766.
Lincoln, K. D., Taylor, R. J., Bullard, M., Chatters, L. M., Woodward, A. T., Himle, J. A., et al. (2010). Emotional support, negative interaction and DSM IV lifetime disorders among older African Americans: Findings from the national survey of American life (NSAL). *International Journal of Geriatric Psychiatry, 25*(6), 612–621.
Link, B. G., & Phelan, J. (1995). Social conditions as fundamental causes of disease. *Journal of Health and Social Behavior, 35*, 80–94.
Luckow, A., Reifman, A., & McIntosh. D. N. (1998). Presented to the annual meeting of the American psychological association. San Francisco.
Lynch, J. J. (1977). *The broken heart*. New York: Basic Books.
Matthews, S., Stansfeld, S., & Power, C. (1999). Social support at age 33: The influence of gender, employment status and social class. *Social Science and Medicine, 49*(1), 133–142.

Mickelson, K. D., & Kubzansky, L. D. (2003). Social distribution of social support: The mediating role of life events. *American Journal of Community Psychology, 32*(3–4), 265–281.

Myers, J. K., Lindenthal, J. J., Pepper, M. P., & Ostrander, D. R. (1972). Life events and mental status: A longitudinal study. *Journal of Health and Social Behavior, 13*(4), 398–406.

Newsom, J. T., Nishishiba, M., Morgan, D. L., & Rook, K. S. (2003). The relative importance of three domains of positive and negative social exchanges: A longitudinal model with comparable measures. *Psychology and Aging, 18*(4), 746–754.

Newsom, J. T., Rook, K. S., Nishishiba, M., Sorkin, D. H., & Mahan, T. L. (2005). Understanding the relative importance of positive and negative social exchanges: Examining specific domains and appraisals. *The Journals of Gerontology. Series B. Psychological Sciences and Social Sciences, 60*(6), 304–312.

Pagel, M. D., Erdly, W. W., & Becker, J. (1987). Social networks: We get by with (and in spite of) a little help from our friends. *Journal of Personality and Social Psychology, 53*(4), 793–804.

Pearlin, L. I. (1989). The sociological study of stress. *Journal of Health and Social Behavior, 30*(3), 241–256.

Pearlin, L. I., Menaghan, E. G., Lieberman, M. A., & Mullan, J. T. (1981). The stress process. *Journal of Health and Social Behavior, 22*(4), 337–356.

Pearlin, L. I., & Schooler, C. (1978). The structure of coping. *Journal of Health and Social Behavior, 19*(1), 2–21.

Reinhardt, J. P. (2001). Effects of positive and negative support received and provided on adaptation to chronic visual impairment. *Applied Developmental Science, 5*(2), 76–85.

Resnick, M. D., et al. (1997). Protecting adolescents from harm: Findings from the national longitudinal study on adolescent health. *JAMA, 278*(10), 823–832.

Revenson, T. A., Schiaffino, K. M., Deborah Majerovitz, S., & Gibofsky, A. (1991). Social support as a double-edged sword: The relation of positive and problematic support to depression among rheumatoid arthritis patients. *Social Science & Medicine, 33*(7), 807–813.

Robles, T. F., & Kiecolt-Glaser, J. K. (2003). The physiology of marriage: Pathways to health. *Physiology & Behavior, 79*(3), 409–416.

Rook, K. S. (1984). The negative side if social interaction: Impact on psychological well-being. *Journal of Personality and Social Psychology, 46*, 1097–1108.

Rook, K. S. (2001). Emotional health and positive versus negative social exchanges: A daily diary analysis. *Applied Developmental Science, 5*(2), 86–97.

Rook, K. S. (2003). Exposure and reactivity to negative social exchanges: A preliminary investigation using daily diary data. *The Journals of Gerontology. Series B, Psychological Sciences and Social Sciences, 58*(2), 100–111.

Rosenberg, M. (1979). *Conceiving the self*. New York: Basic Books.

Rosenberg, M., & McCullough, B. C. (1981). Mattering: Inferred significance and mental health among adolescents. *Research in Community & Mental Health*, 163–182.

Ross, C. E., & Mirowsky, J. (1989). Explaining the social patterns of depression: Control and problem solving–or support and talking? *Journal of Health and Social Behavior, 30*(2), 206–219.

Rowe, J. W., & Kahn, R. L. (1987). Human aging: Usual and successful. *Science, 237*(4811), 143–149.

Ruehlman, L. S., & Karoly, P. (1991). With a little flak from my friends: Development and preliminary validation of the test of negative social exchange (TENSE). *Psychological Assessment: A Journal of Consulting and Clinical Psychology, 3*(1), 97–104.

Ryan, W. (1971). *Blaming the victim*. New York: Pantheon.

Sacco, P., Casado, B. L., & Unick, G. J. (2011). Differential item functioning across race in aging research: An example using a social support measure. *Clinical Gerontologist, 34*(1), 57–70.

Salonna, F., Geckova, A. M., Zezula, I., Sleskova, M., Groothoff, J. W., Reijneveld, S. A., et al. (2012). Does social support mediate or moderate socioeconomic differences in self-rated health among adolescents? *International Journal of Public Health, 57*(3), 609–617.

Sarason, B. A., Pierce, G. R., & Sarason, I. G. (1990). Social support: The sense of acceptance and the role of relationships. In B. R. Sarason, I. G. Sarason, & G. R. Pierce (Eds.), *Social support: An interactional view* (pp. 97–128). New York: Wiley.

Sarason, I. G., & Sarason, B. R. (Eds.). (1985). *Social support: Theory, research and applications*. Boston: Martinus Nijhoff.
Schachter, S. (1959). *The psychology of affiliation: Experimental studies of the sources of gregariousness*. Stanford, CA: Stanford University Press.
Son, J., Lin, N., & George, L. K. (2008). Cross-national comparison of social support structures between Taiwan and the United States. *Journal of Health and Social Behavior, 49*(1), 104–117.
Stafford, M., McMunn, A., Zaninotto, P., & Nazroo, J. (2011). Positive and negative exchanges in social relationships as predictors of depression: Evidence from the English longitudinal study of aging. *Journal of Aging and Health, 23*(4), 607–628.
Stice, E. (2002). Risk and maintenance factors for eating pathology: A meta-analytic review. *Psychological Bulletin, 128*(5), 825–848.
Strogatz, D. S., Croft, J. B., James, S. A., Keenan, N. L., Browning, S. R., Garrett, J. M., et al. (1997). Social support, stress, and blood pressure in black adults. *Epidemiology, 8*(5), 482–487.
Syme, S. L., & Berkman, L. F. (1976). Social class, susceptibility and sickness. *American Journal of Epidemiology, 104*(1), 1–8.
Taylor, S. E., Klein, L. C., Lewis, B. P., Gruenewald, T. L., Gurung, R. A. R., & Updegraff, J. A. (2000). Biobehavioral responses to stress in females: Tend-and-befriend, not fight-or-flight. *Psychological Review, 107*(3), 411–429.
Thoits, P. A. (1995). Stress, coping, and social support processes: Where are we? What next? *Journal of Health and Social Behavior, 35*, 53–79.
Thoits, P. A. (2011). Mechanisms linking social ties and support to physical and mental health. *Journal of Health and Social Behavior, 52*(2), 145–161.
Thomas, W. I., & Thomas, D. S. T. (1928). *The child in America: Behavior problems and programs*. New York: Johnson Reprint Corp.
Turner, R. J. (1983). Direct, indirect and moderating effects of social support upon psychological distress and associated conditions. In H. B. Kaplan (Ed.), *Psychosocial stress: Trends in theory and research* (pp. 105–155). New York: Academic Press.
Turner, H. A. (1994). Gender and social support: Taking the bad with the good? *Sex Roles, 30*, 521–541.
Turner, R. J., & Avison, W. R. (1989). Gender and depression: Assessing exposure and vulnerability to life events in a chronically strained population. *The Journal of Nervous and Mental Disease, 177*(8), 443–455.
Turner, R. J., Brown, T. N., & Hale, W. B. (2012). Antecedents and consequence off personal resources: Evidence on the causation selection debate. Presented at the annual meeting of the American sociological Association, Denver.
Turner, R. J., Frankel, B. G., & Levin, D. M. (1983). Social support: Conceptualization, measurement, and implications for mental health. *Research in Community Mental Health, 3*, 67–111.
Turner, R. J., & Marino, F. (1994). Social support and social structure: A descriptive epidemiology. *Journal of Health and Social Behavior, 35*(3), 193–212.
Turner, R. J., & Noh, S. (1988). Physical disability and depression: A longitudinal analysis. *Journal of Health and Social Behavior, 29*(1), 23–37.
Turner, R. J., Taylor, J., & Van Gundy, K. (2004). Personal resources and depression in the transition to adulthood: Ethnic comparisons. *Journal of Health and Social Behavior, 45*(1), 34–52.
Turner, H. A., & Turner, R. J. (1999). Gender, social status, and emotional reliance. *Journal of Health and Social Behavior, 40*(4), 360–373.
Uchino, B. N., Cacioppo, J. T., & Kiecolt-Glaser, J. K. (1996). The relationship between social support and physiological processes: A review with emphasis on underlying mechanisms and implications for health. *Psychological Bulletin, 119*(3), 488–531.
Umberson, D. (1987). Family status and health behaviors: Social control as a dimension of social integration. *Journal of Health and Social Behavior, 28*(3), 306–319.
Umberson, D., Chen, M. D., House, J. S., Hopkins, K., & Slaten, E. (1996). The effect of social relationships on psychological well-being: Are men and women really so different? *American Sociological Review, 61*(5), 837–857.

Umberson, D., & Montez, J. K. (2010). Social relationships and health a flashpoint for health policy. *Journal of Health and Social Behavior, 51*(1 suppl), S54–S66.

Vaux, A. (1988). *Social support: Theory, research, and intervention*. New York: Praeger.

Vega, W. A., & Miranda, M. R. (1985). *Stress and Hispanic mental health*. Rockville, MD: National Institute of Public Health.

Veil, H. O. F., & Baumann, U. (1992). The many meanings of social support. In H. O. F. Veil & U. Baumann (Eds.), *The meaning and measurement of social support* (pp. 1–7). New York: Hemisphere.

Wethington, E., & Kessler, R. C. (1986). Perceived support, received support, and adjustment to stressful life events. *Journal of Health and Social Behavior, 27*(1), 78–89.

Wethington, E., McLeod, J. D., & Kessler, R. C. (1987). The importance of life events for explaining sex differences in psychological distress. In R. C. Barnett, L. Biener, & G. K. Baruch (Eds.), *Gender*. New York: Free Press.

Wills, T. A., McNamara, G., Vaccaro, D., & Hirky, A. E. (1997). Escalated substance use: A longitudinal grouping analysis from early to muddle adolescence. In G. A. Marlatt & G. R. VandenBos (Eds.), *Addictive behaviors* (pp. 97–128). Washington D.C.: American Psychological Association.

Chapter 2
Twenty Years of the Sociology of Mental Health: The Continued Significance of Gender and Marital Status for Emotional Well-Being

Robin W. Simon

2.1 Introduction

The formation of the Mental Heath Section of the American Sociological Association in 1992 heralded a period of considerable excitement, energy, and creativity in theory and research on the social determinants of mental health. The availability of a new institutional identity had a galvanizing effect on section members, who welcomed greater opportunities for social interaction with scholars working on similar substantive issues and ideas. Two areas in which this wave of enthusiasm and synergy is particularly evident pertain to gender and marital status differences in emotional well-being. Over the past couple of decades, sociologists have made significant theoretical, analytical, and substantive progress in our understanding of *how* and *why* people's gender and marital status—two axes of social inequality in the United States—influence their mental health. Building on theory and research from the 1970s and 1980s, when research on the relationships between gender, marital status, and mental health first gained traction, the last 20 years of scholarship has produced an impressive body of work elucidating a multitude of social—including social structural, social psychological, and socio-cultural—factors that contribute to persistent gender and marital status differences in emotional well-being.

In light of profound social changes in the nature and organization of both gender and marriage that have been evolving in the U.S. since the last quarter of the 20th century, it is not surprising that much of this research compares the emotional consequences of major adult social roles and relationships for women and men. In the last decades of the 20th and first decades of the 21st centuries, women's

---

R.W. Simon (✉)
Wake Forest University, Winston-Salem, North Carolina, USA
e-mail: simonr@wfu.edu

labor force participation was at an all time high as were dual-earner families (Bianchi and Milke 2010). Moreover, although the divorce rate leveled off during this period, it continued to be high as were rates of single-parenthood, remarriage, and non-marital heterosexual cohabitation (Cherlin 2010). Additionally, while an increasing number of women were the primary breadwinners of their families, the recent downturn in the economy led to a growing number of un- or under-employed men—many of whom are husbands and fathers (Cherlin 2010). On top of changes in men's and women's social roles and relationships, the revolution in longevity has resulted in an increase in the proportion of older adults in the population living as both couples and single persons; cultural shifts in Americans' views about homosexuality have also led to a recent upsurge of men and women who are openly in same-sex intimate relationships—many of which involve minor children (Powell et al. 2010). A result of these and other social changes is that there is an unprecedented number of men and women in the U.S. today living outside of traditional marriage that includes an employed husband/father, a homemaker wife/mother, and the minor children they had together; the 2010 Census indicates that less than one-third of all American households represent this type of family (United States Census Bureau 2010).

Armed with an arsenal of high quality data, sophisticated analytic techniques, and nuanced hypotheses based on insights from several substantive areas within sociology and cognate disciplines, sociologists of mental health have been shedding light on how men and women are coping with these new social forms and arrangements. The past 20 years of research reveals that while some of these social changes have created new opportunities for men and women and are associated with increased emotional well-being, others are highly stressful and detrimental for their mental health. Indeed, the stress process paradigm—which focuses on the mediating and moderating role of personal resources such as financial and psychosocial resources including social support—continues to be the dominant framework for explaining observed gender and marital status differences in mental health. At the same time, researchers have been paying closer attention to the larger social, economic, and cultural context in which men and women's lives are embedded, the proximate social conditions under which their social roles and relationships are emotionally beneficial or harmful as well as the different ways they express mental health problems. By identifying macro- and meso-level social causes of micro-level emotional processes, this new wave of research on gender and marital status disparities in mental health exemplifies the unique strength of the sociological perspective.

In this chapter, I summarize some broad themes that have emerged over the past two decades of scholarship on gender, marital status, and mental health, broadly defined—highlighting important theoretical continuities and new developments, methodological innovations as well as key substantive findings. However, because these are highly prolific areas of scholarship, I will not discuss all studies on these separate yet highly interrelated topics that have appeared in print since the early 1990s. A recent count indicates that 45 articles on gender and mental health, and another 32 articles on marriage and mental health, have been published in the *Journal of Health and Social Behavior* between 1992 and 2012; many more articles have appeared in other specialty sociology and health journals—including the new section journal *Society and Mental Health, Social Science and Medicine, Journal of Marriage and Family, Gender and Society, Social Psychology Quarterly* as well as sociology's generalist journals such as the *American Journal of Sociology, American Sociological Review, Social Forces*, and *Social Problems*. My review is, therefore, highly selective and reflects my own idiosyncratic scholarly interests in gender variation in the emotional impact of adult social roles and relationships—particularly work and family roles and intimate (including, but not limited to, marital) relationships. In addition to taking stock of what we have learned about these status inequalities in emotional well-being since the formation of the ASA Mental Health section, I discuss some promising new directions for theory and research that would further social science knowledge about the continued significance of gender and marital status for mental health during this historical period of social change.

2.2 Twenty Years of Theory and Research on Gender, Marital Status, and Mental Health

2.2.1 Gender and Emotional Well-Being

One of the most vexing social problems that has long preoccupied sociologists of gender and mental health is that women have higher rates of depressive disorders than men. Recent epidemiological studies based on non-clinical populations of adults indicate that women are twice as likely as men to experience this mental health problem (Kessler 2003). Moreover, the gender gap in depressive disorder has been fairly stable over the past four decades (Dohrenwend and Dohrenwend 1977; Weissman and Klerman 1977) despite greater educational and employment opportunities for women since the last quarter of the 20th century along with their more expansive roles in the family, workplace, and society, women continue to meet criteria for affective disorders at a rate that is double that of men's. The female excess of depression in the adult population is an intractable social problem that has both personal and society-wide impacts; not only is it the leading cause of disease-related disability among women but it is associated with a host of other social and economic consequences for themselves, their families, and their communities (World Health Organization 2000).

Decades of sociological research based on community and national surveys have produced similar results for self-reports of depressive symptoms in the general population of adults; in most studies conducted from the 1970s to the present, women report significantly more symptoms of depression than men (Rosenfield and Mouzon 2013). Recognizing that depression is only one of many dimensions of emotional distress (see Simon 2007 for a review), researchers over the past two decades have also assessed gender differences in the experience of a variety of everyday emotions. Paralleling findings for depressed affect, these studies reveal that women report significantly more frequent negative emotions including anger as well as significantly fewer positive emotions such as happiness than do men (Ross and Van Willigen 1996; Simon and Nath 2004; Simon and Lively 2010; Stevenson and Wolfers 2009, but also see Yang 2008 for an exception). The gender gap in these indicators of emotional distress represents a challenging paradox for gender and mental health scholars across many disciplines who assumed there would be greater gender parity in mental health as women's social roles and relationships began to resemble those of men.

Sociologists have developed three main hypotheses about this mental health disparity. The first is the exposure hypothesis, the second is the vulnerability hypothesis, and the third and most recent is the gendered-response hypothesis. These hypotheses differ with respect to the etiology of women's greater emotional distress—including the structure and nature of their social roles and relationships, the personal resources they are able to mobilize in the face of life stress as well as the ways in which they express emotional upset relative to men.

2.2.1.1 The Exposure Hypothesis: Women are More Exposed than Men to Role-Related Stress

It is now 40 years since (Gove 1972; Gove and Tudor 1973) introduced his highly influential sex-role theory of mental illness that argues that the higher rate of emotional disturbance among women in the U.S. is due to their roles in society, which are presumably less satisfying and more stressful than are men's. Gove attributed women's relatively greater distress to their role as homemaker, which he claimed is a restrictive, socially isolating, and devalued social position that offers modern women little opportunity for self-fulfillment, social interaction with other adults, and financial independence. In contrast, men's social roles are expansive, interesting and self-affirming, providing greater financial rewards, adult interaction, and marital power. While he recognized that combining employment with marriage and parenthood is likely be more stressful for women than men, the implication of Gove's sex-role theory is that women's mental health would improve once their social roles and relationships were more like men's.

Gove's seminal insights were the catalyst for much empirical research on gender and mental health in the 1970s and 1980s, which I noted earlier was a period marked by the steady rise in female employment—particularly the employment of wives and mothers. Much of this research compared the mental health of men and women who hold similar numbers and types of roles, especially the roles of spouse, parent, and worker. In essence, these studies evaluated the *exposure hypothesis*, which posits that gender inequality in mental health is due to gender inequality in exposure to role-related stress. Interestingly, this research produced equivocal findings with respect to the emotional benefits of employment among married women; for example, while some studies found no distress differences between employed wives and homemakers (Aneshensel et al. 1981; Cleary and Mechanic 1983; Gore and Magione 1983; Pearlin 1975), others showed that employed wives are significantly less distressed than their non-employed peers (Kessler and McRae 1982; Rosenfield 1980). Findings were, however, unequivocal with respect to differences in psychological well-being between men and women in dual-earner families; in numerous studies, employed wives reported significantly more symptoms of psychological distress than their male counterparts (Kessler and McRae 1982; Menaghan 1989; Rosenfield 1980; Thoits 1986). Another interesting finding from this body of work is that husbands of employed wives reported significantly more distress than husbands of homemakers (Kessler and McRae 1982; Rosenfield 1980, 1992; Ross et al. 1983).

Sociological research on gender and mental health over the past two decades has continued to evaluate the exposure hypothesis but in contrast to earlier studies, recent studies have gone beyond comparisons of the well-being of women and men who hold the same configurations of social statuses. This research focuses on elucidating the larger *social conditions* under which combining work and family roles is more or less stressful and distressing for women and men. Scholars have identified a number of social structural factors that contribute to women's greater distress in dual-earner families. Wives' relatively lower incomes, limited access to high quality, affordable child-care outside the home as well as husbands' failure to participate more equitably in the division of household labor have emerged as pivotal structural factors that contribute to the persistence of gender inequality in emotional well-being in these families (Bird 1999; Glass and Fugimoto 1994; Lennon and Rosenfield 1995; Lively et al. 2010; Ross and Mirowsky 1988; Ross et al. 1983). Although the gender gap in time spent in paid and non-paid work has narrowed over the past two decades (Bianchi et al. 2007), a recent study shows that multitasking—more common among mothers than fathers in dual-earner families—is a continued source of chronic strain, negative emotions, and psychological distress for working mothers (Offer and Schneider 2011). Hochschild's (1989) formative work on dual-earner families shows that wives' perceived inequity in the division of household labor between themselves and their husbands, and the unpleasant interpersonal dynamics and emotions it gives rise to, not only have negative consequences for their mental health but also for marital quality.

Other studies find that social psychological factors such as women's low sense of control, particularly in the face of high work and family demands, also help explain the gender gap in depressive symptoms among employed spouses residing with minor children (Lennon and Rosenfield 1995; Rosenfield 1992). A sense of powerless to alter the structurally unequal and subsequently stressful situations to which they are disproportionately exposed plays an etiological role in employed wives' poorer mental health as well (Lennon and Rosenfield 1995; Simon and Lively 2010). Still other research reveals that sociocultural factors—including gendered beliefs about men's and women's work and family identities—also contribute to male-female differences in well-being. For example, I found that a reason why combing work and family is less advantageous for women's than men's mental health is because work and family roles have fundamentally different meanings for the genders; whereas men's family roles are based on the provision of economic support to their families, employment detracts from women's ability to provide care and nurturance to their spouse and children (Simon 1995, 1997). The emotional benefits of combining work and family identities are greater for men than for women because employment contributes to men's identity as a "good" father and husband but interferes with women's identity as a "good" mother and wife.

In short, while social change in women's social roles and relationships has created greater opportunities for themselves and their families, it has also been met with some new forms of structural inequality, which are both stressful and distressing. The failure of husbands to engage more fully in the home, wives' relatively lower incomes, the lack of high quality affordable child-care outside the home as well as deeply held cultural beliefs about the nature and meaning of men's and women's family identities continue to play a pivotal role in employed married mothers relatively higher levels of emotional distress. However, while I focused on gender differences in mental health in dual-earner marriages, research also indicates that the stress women experience from combining work and family roles is even greater in families in which they are single-parents (Avison et al. 2007; McLanahan 1983; Simon 1998). This finding suggests that the gender gap in emotional well-being may be even greater among non-married than among married employed parents—a point to which I return in the section on marital status and mental health.

Although this body of research clearly indicates that gender inequality in exposure to certain types of stressors helps explain gender inequality in emotional distress, sociologists recognize that there is no single explanation of the complex and seemingly intractable disparities in mental health. That is, structurally based gender inequality in the family and workplace are necessary but not sufficient for explaining the persistence of women's greater distress. To more fully understand the gender gap in mental health, sociologists have turned to the *vulnerability hypothesis*, which posits that women are also more vulnerable than men to the adverse emotional effects of stress.

2.2.1.2 The Vulnerability Hypothesis: Women are More Vulnerable than Men to the Impact of Stress

Pearlin and Schooler (1978), Kessler (1979a), and Thoits (1982) were among the first to argue that members of socially disadvantaged groups in the U.S. are not only more exposed to life stress but also possess fewer personal resources, which enhance emotional well-being as well as reduce (i.e., buffer) the negative impact of stressful life circumstances. Whereas the exposure hypothesis locates the etiology of psychological distress in structurally-based social inequality, the vulnerability hypothesis attributes disparities in mental health to the *social psychology of inequality*—particularly inequality in the possession of psychosocial resources. With respect to gender, these and other scholars surmised that women's insufficient social support and coping resources (a by-product of structural gender inequality) renders them more vulnerable or reactive than men to the psychological impact of both acute and chronic stressors; women's greater stress-reactivity, in turn, helps explain their relatively poorer mental health. In his influential study using a novel analytic technique, Kessler (1979b) found that differential impact is a more important determinant of the relationships between gender and distress than differential exposure.

Sociological research over the past several decades investigated gender differences in personal resources and psychological vulnerability, though with mixed results. Studies consistently find that men and women have different coping styles and strategies for dealing with stress. For example, while men tend to have an inexpressive coping style and are more likely to control their emotions, women tend to have an emotional and emotionally expressive style of coping (Simon and Nath 2004; Thoits 1991). These studies also show that men are more likely to use problem-focused coping strategies, whereas women are more likely to use emotion-focused coping and seek social support. Additionally, a large body of work documents gender differences in perceptions of control (or mastery), which also play an important role in gender differences in mental health (Mirowsky and Ross 2006; Thoits 1991, 1995). As I noted earlier, studies indicate that women's low sense of control in the face of high demands from combining work and family responsibilities contribute to the gender gap in depressive symptoms in dual-earner families (Lennon and Rosenfield 1995; Rosenfield 1989). Women's lower sense of personal control no doubt reflects their continued unequal status, power, and resources in the family, workplace, and larger society (see Simon and Lively 2010).

Interestingly, research is somewhat more equivocal with respect to gender differences in self-esteem. While some researchers find little evidence of women's lower self-esteem (Miller and Kirsh 1989; Thoits 1995)—which may be a positive outcome of women's increasingly expansive role in the workplace, family, and society—others show that women continue to report lower self-esteem than do men (McMullin and Cairney 2004; Robins and Trzesniewski 2005; Rosenfield and Mouzon 2013; Thoits 2010; Turner and Marino 1994; Turner and Roszell Turner 1994). At the same time, however, women report more rather than less social support than men (Thoits 1995; Turner and Marino 1994; Turner and Turner 1999). Moreover, despite the abundance of studies documenting that efficacious coping resources and perceived social support reduce the negative impact of eventful and chronic stressors (Thoits 1982, 1987; Turner and Turner 1999), gender differences in the possession of psychosocial resources do not explain gender differences in emotional distress (see Aneshensel 1992 and Thoits 1995, 2010 for reviews).

Additionally, with the exception of Turner et al. (1995) study, which finds greater female vulnerability to the depressive effects of acute and chronic stress, there is little evidence that women are more vulnerable than men *in general* (Aneshensel et al. 1991; Lennon 1987; Newman 1986; Simon 1998; Turner and Avison 1989). Rather, studies reveal that certain stressors are more distressing for women and others are more distressing for men. While women tend to be more reactive to family-related and interpersonal stress, men tend to be more reactive to employment-related stress (Conger et al. 1993; Pearlin and Lieberman 1979; Kessler and McLeod 1984; Simon 1992, 1998, Simon and Robin 2000; Simon and Lively 2010 but also see Ensinger and Celentano 1990, Lennon 1987, and Newman 1986 for exceptions with respect to the greater impact of work-related stress on men). Scholars have attributed these findings to gender socialization that begins in childhood as well as the different adult role-responsibilities that are socially assigned to women and men. By continuing to hold men responsible for their family's economic support, and women responsible for providing nurturance to loved ones and maintaining interpersonal relationships within and outside the family, it is reasonable to conclude that stress in work and family domains differentially effect the well-being of women and men.

Taking these findings one-step further, Thoits (1991, 1992) argues that stressors may not have the same meaning and emotional significance for the genders; stressors that threaten peoples' valued identities and self-concepts (i.e., identity-relevant stressors) are more harmful for mental health than identity-irrelevant stressors. These important insights suggest that observed gender differences in vulnerability to work and family-related stress reflect differences in the salience of work and family identities for women and men. In support of this argument, I found that the impact of children's health and behavior problems on emotional distress is greater for mothers than fathers because the parental identity is more important for women's self-conception than it is for men's (Simon 1992). Gender differences in vulnerability to work and family stress also depend on marital status, which alters the meaning of work and family roles for women and men. For example, in a study that included symptoms of both depression and substance abuse, I found that married mothers are more vulnerable than married fathers to chronic marital and parental strain, but married fathers are more vulnerable than married mothers to the effects of financial strain (Simon 1998). There were, however, no gender differences in the impact of financial strain among unmarried parents; moreover, unmarried fathers were more rather than less vulnerable to parental strain than their female peers. These findings indicate that *marital status* is an important part of the *social context* that shapes the meaning and emotional significance of work and family roles and identities for women and men. One further point: These complex patterns of male and female vulnerability were evident for symptoms of depression among women and symptoms of substance problems among men.

Indeed, in her seminal work on differential vulnerability, Aneshensel (1992, Aneshensel et al. 1991) argued that gender differences in stress-reactivity are highly specific and depend not only on the stressor involved but also on the mental health problem considered. She notes that because most studies are based on mental health problems that are more common among women (i.e., symptoms of depression and generalized distress) and do not include those that are more common among men (e.g., antisocial behavior and substance abuse/dependence), they tend to *over*estimate female vulnerability and distress and *under*estimate men's. Aneshensel's theoretical insights are the basis for the third major hypothesis about the relationship between gender and mental health.

In sum, the past several decades of research on gender and mental health have produced inconsistent but nonetheless important results regarding gender inequality in both the possession of psychosocial resources and psychological vulnerability. In contrast to earlier claims that women's insufficient coping and social support render them more vulnerable to the deleterious emotional consequences of stress in general, it appears that some stressors are more distressing for women while others are more distressing for men. The stressors that are most harmful for men and women tend to be those in role domains for which they are responsible. However, while theory and research on differential vulnerability has expanded our knowledge about social psychological factors that mediate and moderate the relationship between sex, stress, and distress, the vulnerability hypothesis does not explain persistent gender differences in mental health.

2.2.1.3 The Gendered-Response Hypothesis: Men and Women Express Distress and Respond to Stress with Different Types of Mental Health Problems

The inability of the vulnerability hypothesis to account for the gender gap in mental health led to the development of the third main hypothesis about the relationship between sex, stress, and psychological distress. Over the past two decades, sociologists have increasingly turned their attention to the *gendered-response hypothesis*, which argues that women are not more distressed and vulnerable than men, but that males and females express emotional distress and respond to stress with different and gendered-types of psychological problems. Animated by Aneshensel's (1992) (Aneshensel et al. 1991) pivotal insights about the highly specific ways in which stress affects women and men, researchers have been examining the effects of different stressors on a range of mental health problems— including those that are commonly found among men. As I noted above, the failure of studies to examine male-typical expressions of psychological disturbance has resulted in overestimates women's distress and psychological vulnerability and underestimates of men's. As their starting point, advocates of the gendered-response hypothesis point to epidemiological estimates of rates of specific types of mental health problems among men and women in the U.S.

Epidemiological research on both lifetime and recent prevalence rates of mental disorders conducted from the 1970s to the present consistently document that although women have higher rates of affective and anxiety disorders (and their psychological corollaries of symptoms of non-specific distress, anxiety, and depression), men have higher rates of antisocial personality and substance abuse/dependence disorders (and their psychological corollaries of antisocial behavior and symptoms of substance abuse/dependence) (Dohrenwend and Dohrenwend 1977; Meyers et al. 1984; Robins and Regier 1994; Kessler et al. 1993, 1994). Interestingly, research on adolescent mental health conducted over the past two decades also documents gender differences in these mental health problems; studies that compare boys' and girls' emotional well-being reveal that by mid- to late-adolescence, girls report significantly more symptoms of depression, whereas boys report significantly more symptoms of antisocial behavior and substance problems (Avison and McAlpine 1992; Gore et al. 1992; Rosenfield 1999a, b). Hagan and Foster's (2003) study provides insight into gendered pathways or trajectories of mental health problems from early adolescence to emerging adulthood; based on the National Longitudinal Study of Adolescent Health, they find that angry emotions experienced in early adolescence—a result of stressful family circumstances—increase the likelihood of rebellious or aggressive behavior in middle adolescence and the development of depressive symptoms among females and substance problems among males in young adulthood. In other words, males and females tend to respond to a similarly stressful childhood situation with different mental health problems as adults.

On the basis of these and other studies (including the National Co-Morbidity Studies, Kessler et al. 1993), mental health scholars agree that although there are gender differences in the prevalence of specific types of mental disorders, there are no gender differences in the *overall* prevalence of mental health problems (see Rosenfield and Mouzon 2013 and Simon 2007 for reviews). Females tend to manifest distress and respond to stress with *internalizing* problems such as depression, whereas males are more likely to express emotional disturbance and react to stress with *externalizing* problems including antisocial behavior and substance abuse/dependence. Because gender differences in rates of these specific types of problems are evident in adolescence—years before males and females acquire adult social roles—sociologists of mental health now argue that we cannot continue to attribute male-female differences in mental health in adulthood solely to differences in the structure and meaning of men's and women's adult roles.

The past 20 years of research provides empirical support for the gendered-response hypothesis. An accumulating body of work (including Hagan and Foster's 2003 study) reveals that the impact of some types of stress does not differ for men and women when gendered expressions of distress are considered. Much of this work is based on longitudinal analyses of the mental health consequences of marital-status transitions for women and men. Several studies indicate that while women tend to respond to the stress associated with divorce and widowhood with elevated symptoms of depression, men tend to respond to these same sources of stress with increases in symptoms of substance problems (Horwitz et al. 1996; Simon 2002; Umberson et al. 1996; Williams 2003). These studies also find that the emotional benefits associated with becoming married accrue to women and men; the transition to marriage (and remarriage) significantly reduces depressive symptoms among women and substance problems among men. These findings are consistent with epidemiological research as well as Aneshensel's (1992) argument about gender differences in stress-reactivity. They are not, however, consistent with Gove's early sex-role theory of mental illness that I discussed earlier (1972), which posits that marriage improves men's emotional well-being but harms women's (also see Bernard 1982).

In addition to studies that reveal no gender difference in vulnerability to these types of eventful stressors, studies find no gender difference in the mental health impact of certain types of chronic stress. In an earlier study, Lennon (1987) found that stressful job characteristics—including a lack of control, autonomy, and creativity in one's occupation—are associated with more depressive symptoms among women and substance problems among men. Although women disproportionately find themselves in jobs that have these emotionally unhealthy characteristics (Roxburgh 1996), neither men nor women are more vulnerable to emotional effects of this source of chronic stress.

However, other studies document gender differences in vulnerability to other types of chronic stress—even when gender-typical expressions of distress are examined. As I noted above, one of my earlier studies showed that the association between both marital and parental strain with depressive symptoms is greater for married women than married men, but there is no gender difference in the association between these sources of stress and substance problems among the married (Simon 1998). In contrast, although there is no gender difference in the association between financial strain and depressive symptoms among the married, the association between this source of stress and substance abuse is greater for married men than married women. In a more recent study, Simon and Barrett (2010) found that certain dimensions of non-marital romantic relationships in early adulthood are differentially associated with young men's and women's mental health. Status dimensions of these relationships (e.g., being in a current romantic relationship and a recent romantic breakup) are more depressing for women than for men, whereas dimensions of an on-going relationship (i.e., partner support and strain) have a greater impact on symptoms of alcohol problems among men. Together, these findings indicate that certain stressors do *not* equally affect the mental health of women and men.

Not surprisingly, sociologists have developed provocative and compelling explanations of why males and females tend to express emotional upset and respond to stress with different types of mental health problems. Drawing on insights from sociological social psychology and cognitive psychology, Rosenfield attributes gendered-expressions of distress to gender-differentiated structures of the self (or self-schemas) that develop in adolescence. She argues that a result of female socialization in childhood—which emphasizes the importance of others for self-development—is that females tend to develop an "other-focused" self that privileges the collective over the self in social relations. In contrast, a result of male socialization in childhood—which emphasizes the importance of independence for self-development—is that the males tend to develop an "ego-focused" self that privileges the self over others in social relations. In a systematic program of research on adolescents and emerging adults (Rosenfield et al. 2000, 2005, 2006), she finds that these different self-schema increase the risk of different types of mental health problems; persons with other-salience schema (i.e., adolescent girls) are predisposed to internalizing problems including depression, while those with self-salient schema (i.e., adolescent boys) are predisposed to externalizing problems such as antisocial behavior and substance abuse. She also demonstrates that gender differences in self- and other-salience mediate gender differences in internalizing and externalizing mental health problems.

It is worth noting that the concepts of self- and other-salience closely correspond to the concepts of agency and communion, which have long been discussed in the literature on gendered personality (e.g., Parsons 1955). Although its not yet been tested, gender differences in self- and other-salience may also help explain why "self-events" (i.e., undesirable events that occur to oneself) tend to be more distressing for men, whereas "other-events" (i.e., negative events that occur to people in one's social network) tend to be more distressing for women (Aneshensel et al. 1991; Kessler and McLeod 1984; Turner and Avison 1989). Future research testing these ideas should, of course, include male and female typical expressions of distress.

Viewing these observed gendered-patterns of distress and vulnerability through a somewhat different though closely-related lens, I attribute gender differences in rates of internalizing and externalizing mental health problems to the larger emotional culture of the U.S. and gender-linked norms about the appropriate experience and expression of emotion for males and females (Simon 2000, 2002, 2007; Simon and Nath 2004). Drawing on theoretical insights from the sociologies of gender and emotion, I argue that embodied in Americans' emotional culture are beliefs about the "proper" emotional styles of males and females as well as emotion norms that specify "appropriate" feeling and expression for men and women (also see Hochschild 1979, 1983, Smith-Lovin 1995; and Thoits 1989). Because feelings of depression signal weakness to self and others—and weakness is a permissible personality characteristic for females but not for males in the U.S.—it is an acceptable emotion for females but a sanctioned emotion for males. A consequence of gender-linked emotional socialization throughout the life course is that females learn to express emotional upset with internalizing emotional problem including depression, while males learn to express distress vis-a`-vis externalizing emotional problems such as substance abuse. Men's higher rate of substance problems reflects their tendency to manage (i.e., suppress) culturally inappropriate feelings of depression with mood-altering substances in order to avoid being labeled "weak" by others and one-self.

However, while the gendered-response hypothesis begins to unravel the complex set of social factors that contribute to sex differences in both the experience and expression of emotional upset, other factors also appear to be involved in the female excess of depressed affect. Recently, Simon and Lively (2010) argued that intense and persistent subjectively experienced anger—more common among women than among men—play a role in their higher levels of depression. Although most sociologists of mental health have focused on anger as an outcome of women's social disadvantage (Mabry and Kiecolt 2005; Ross and Van Willigen 1996), our study showed that anger mediates the relationship between sex and depressive symptoms. In other words, women's more intense and persistent anger—an emotional response to their unfair and unequal work and family roles and relationships—also help explain their higher level of depression relative to men.

Before leaving the topic of gendered-responses to stress, it is important to mention that sociologists are also beginning to examine the links between male and female typical mental health problems and male and female typical physical health problems. A recent study (Needham and Hill 2010) showed that internalizing emotional problems are closely associated with chronic health conditions such as arthritis, headaches, and seasonal allergies, which more common among women. In contrast, externalizing mental health problems are closely associated with life threatening health conditions such as stroke, heart disease, and high blood pressure, which are more common among men. This study also revealed that gender differences in the expression of emotional upset help explain gender differences in physical health problems.

In sum, research that includes male and female typical expressions of distress is a corrective to research that focused exclusively on mental health problems that are more common among females. An examination of internalizing and externalizing emotional problems in tandem allows researchers to assess the degree to which females are more, less, or similarly distressed relative to males. This approach also allows researchers to identify those stressors that have a greater impact on males, those that have a greater impact on females as well as those that take an equal toll on males' and females' mental health. As such, the gendered-response hypothesis—and the body of research evaluating its efficacy—offers a richer and more nuanced picture of the relationship between sex, stress, and psychological distress than either the exposure or vulnerability hypotheses. The socialization experiences of males and females—and the cultural (including emotion) norms upon which gender socialization is based—play an important role in persistent gender differences in mental health.

2.2.1.4 What Have We Learned About Gender and Mental Health Over the Past Two Decades?

Taken together, research on gender and mental health conducted over the past 20 years has made significant progress in our understanding of the social determinants of emotional well-being and gender differences therein. The culmination of research evaluating the exposure, vulnerability, and gendered-response hypotheses indicates that social structural, social psychological, and sociocultural factors are *all* involved in gender differences in mental health. The persistence of gender inequality in the workplace and family continues to play a role in the gender gap in mental health. However, to the extent that current cohorts of women continue to define themselves first and foremost as nurturers and caregivers, and current cohorts of men continue to define themselves primarily as breadwinners, structural changes that have occurred in male's and female's social roles and relationships alone will not produce greater parity in mental health. A focus on emotional well-being reveals that while some aspects of men's and women's lives have changed dramatically over the past decades, other aspects have remained essentially the same.

Two decades ago, Hochschild (1989) referred to this phenomenon as the "stalled revolution" and findings from the past 20 years of research is consistent with this idea. Changes in attitudes about gendered practices in the family have not kept pace with structural changes in the economy. More recently, Gerson (2011) refers to this phenomenon as the "unfinished revolution." Her qualitative research on young men and women indicates that they have more egalitarian views about work and family roles and identities than their parents; current cohorts of young men and women embrace the reality that they will have to combine employment with parenthood and expect to share work and family responsibilities with their future partners. However, Gerson notes that unless there are fundamental changes in workplace that would allow men and women to *balance* employment with parental responsibilities, young women will also experience more stress from combining work and family than young men.

Ridgeway (2011) offers a more theoretical and admittedly even less sanguine account of this contradiction in women's lives—an account that emphasizes the social psychology of gender, particularly the role of deeply entrenched cultural beliefs about women and men. She argues that despite structural changes that have paved the way for gender equality, nominal differences between men and women become infused with traditional gendered beliefs, which in turn maintain and reproduce gendered expectations and practices in both the workplace and family. Whether the recent downturn in the economy, which has disproportionately affected men, will fuel traditional gender beliefs or marshal in a shift in beliefs about men's and women's social roles is currently unknown but is a worthy topic for future research on gender and mental health.

2.2.1.5 Some Current Gaps in Knowledge About Gender and Mental Health

While the past 20 years of scholarship has made significant inroads into our understanding of an array of social factors underlying persistent gender differences in mental health, there are nevertheless several important gaps in knowledge about the relationship between sex, stress, and psychological distress. Page limitations preclude me from discussing all issues that need more scholarly attention so I will touch on what I consider to be two of the most pressing gaps.

The first is that we currently do not know whether the gendered patterns of distress and vulnerability I discussed are evident in minority populations in the U.S. Most studies of gender and mental health have been based on the general population of adults (and more recently adolescents and emerging adults) and have not assessed the degree to which gender inequality interacts with other axes of social inequality to produce different gendered patterns of distress among minorities. Sociologists have increasingly called for an "intersectional" approach to gender research that considers the ways in which race, ethnicity, socioeconomic status, age, and sexual orientation shape the life experiences of males and females. In response to this call, researchers have been examining the intersection of gender, race, and class for mental health (Rosenfield et al. 2006, Rosenfield 2012), gender and mental health over the life course (Barrett 2005; Caputo and Simon 2013; Mirowsky 1996) as well as gender differences in the mental health impact of LBGTQ sexual identities (Ueno 2010); this research has produced interesting results. For example, in a study that included male and female typical mental health problems, Ueno (2010) finds that emerging awareness of same-sex attraction in late adolescence is more distressing for young women than for young men. There has not, however, been much research on gender differences in exposure and vulnerability to work and family stress among African, Hispanic, and Asian Americans. The lack of research on this issue is surprising since there may be greater gender equality in mental health among some minority groups and greater gender inequality in mental health among other minority groups than among white Americans.

As a case in point, our nation's legacy of discrimination against African American men resulted in higher unemployment rates among black men and higher employment rates among black women than their white counterparts throughout the 20th century. A consequence of their shared history of social inequality and disadvantage is that African American men and women tend to have less traditional views about gender and the division of household labor than their white peers (Hill and Sprague 1999; Ladner 1995). It is, therefore, possible that the gender difference in distress and vulnerability in today's dual-earner families is narrower among blacks than among whites. Conversely, because they adhere to more traditional views about gender, the gender difference in distress and vulnerability may be greater among Hispanics and members of lower socioeconomic status groups than among whites and members of higher socioeconomic status groups. We will not know the answer to these and other questions until more mental health research takes an intersectional approach to the study of human health. Springer et al. (2012) recent special issue of *Social Science and Medicine* devoted to this topic represents a positive first step in this direction. Because norms about the "appropriate" experience and expression of emotion may vary by race, ethnicity, age, socioeconomic status, and sexual orientation, studies investigating variations in the relationship between sex, stress, and distress should include multiple—including both mental and physical—indicators of health.

The second important gap in knowledge is that we currently do not know the degree to which potential biological predispositions of males and females are involved in gender differences in emotional distress and vulnerability. Without going into details, recent research in neuroendocrinology and psychophysiology indicates that there is a biological basis for gender differences in anger, depression, and substance abuse (see Simon and Lively 2010 for a brief review). Scholars who study the biology of emotion also recognize that biological factors interact in complex ways with social factors to produce distinct mental health trajectories for males and females. However, while there has been increase in genetics informed sociology, which examines the joint influence of social and genetic factors on happiness and alcohol dependence (Schnittker 2008; Pescosolido et al. 2008), sociologists have been noticeably (and understandably) silent about the potential ways that biology interacts with social circumstances to produce sex differences in mental health (however, see Bird and Rieker 1999; Rieker and Bird 2008; Hopcroft and Bradley 2007; Simon and Lively 2010; and Springer et al. 2012 for exceptions). Fausto-Sterling (1992), an eminent feminist biologist, argues that the failure to acknowledge the complex interactions between the biological and social environment impedes scientific understanding of sex and gender. Sociological research that focuses on the interplay between biological and social factors would expand our knowledge about the relationships between sex, stress, and mental health. As a start, an examination of whether transgender individuals express emotional distress and vulnerability in ways that are consistent with their current or former gender may shed light on the interplay of biological and social factors that shape mental health. Of course, research on members of this highly vulnerable social group must also take into account the stigma and discrimination to which they are routinely exposed.

2.2.2 Marital Status and Emotional Well-Being

In addition to the abundance of sociological theory and research on the relationship between gender and mental health, sociologists have produced an extensive and rich body of theoretical and empirical work on the relationship between marital status and mental health. In fact, one of the most consistent and oft-cited findings from the sociology of mental health since the 1970s is that marriage is associated with significantly higher levels of emotional well-being. This robust finding is evident in community and national samples, cross-sectional and longitudinal analyses, across a variety of household types as well as for several dimensions of mental health. In dozens of studies, married individuals report less emotional distress than their non-married counterparts.

While earlier studies focused on marital status differences in symptoms of depression and non-specific psychological distress (Kessler and McRae 1984; Marks and Lambert 1998; Pearlin and Johnson 1977; Thoits 1986), the past two decades of research on this topic has expanded its focus to include other dimensions of mental health—including substance problems as well as negative and positive affect. This research documents that in addition to reporting significantly fewer symptoms of depression and generalized distress, the married report significantly less substance problems, less frequent negative emotions including anger as well as more frequent positive emotions such as happiness than non-married persons (Caputo and Simon 2013; Simon 2002; Simon and Nath 2004; Umberson et al. 1996; Williams 2003). Marital status differences in emotional well-being in the U.S parallel epidemiological studies, which find lower prevalence rates of psychiatric disorders among married than non-married adults (Williams et al. 1992).

Although these patterns are unequivocal, the direction of the marital status-mental health association has long been a topic of debate; while most sociologists agree that social causation is responsible for married persons' greater emotional well-being, some concede that social selection may underlie the link between marital status and mental health. In contrast to the social causation hypothesis, which argues that marriage improves mental health, the social selection hypothesis posits that persons who enjoy better mental health are more likely than less emotionally healthy persons to become married in the first place; they are also less likely than their less emotionally healthy counterparts to become divorced. However, because they tended to be based on cross-sectional data, earlier studies on this topic were unable to adjudicate between these two competing hypotheses of the relationship between marriage and mental health.

2.2.2.1 Social Causation or Social Selection?—Marital Transitions and Mental Health

Over the past 20 years, sociologists have evaluated the social causation and selection hypotheses by assessing the degree to which marital status transitions result in *changes* in mental health. This research also examines whether individuals' prior mental health predicts marital status change. Several longitudinal studies find that becoming married (and remarried) results in a significant decrease in symptoms of depression and substance abuse, whereas becoming divorced and widowed results in a significant increase in these symptoms of distress (Barrett 2000; Booth and Amato 1991; Marks and Lambert 1998; Simon 2002; Umberson et al. 1996; Williams 2003). These findings clearly support the social causation hypothesis of the relationship between marital status and mental health. At the same time, there is also some support for the social selection argument with respect to marital loss. For example, based on national data, I found that although prior mental health does not predict selection into marriage, persons who reported more symptoms of depression and alcohol abuse were significantly more likely to experience a subsequent divorce than persons who reported lower levels of these symptoms of distress (Simon 2002). These and other findings (Forthofer et al. 1996; Mastekaasa 1992; Menaghan 1985; Wade and Pevalin 2004) indicate that complex social causation and selection processes are *both* involved in the relationship between marriage and mental health.

The past two decades of research on the mental health impact of marital status transitions also sheds light on another issue that has long captured the attention of sociologists: that is, whether the emotional advantage of marriage is greater for men than for women. In contrast to Gove's (1973) early sex-role theory of mental illness, which argues that marriage is advantageous for men but disadvantageous for women (also see Bernard 1982), an accumulating body of work indicates that the advantage of becoming married and disadvantage of becoming divorced and widowed are evident among men and women when gender-typical expressions of distress are considered. The positive impact of marriage and remarriage, and the negative impact of divorce and widowhood, tends to show up in depressive symptoms among women and substance problems among men (Horwitz et al. 1996; Simon 2002; Umberson et al. 1996; Williams 2003). My study further revealed that there are no gender differences in selection into or out of marriage on the basis of prior mental health (Simon 2002). In other words, emotionally robust women are neither more nor less likely to become or remain married than their male peers.

2.2.2.2 Current Explanations of the Mental Health Advantage of Marriage

Why does marriage have positive effects on adults' mental health? For over a century, sociologists have attributed this pattern to a multiplicity of social factors. In his classic study of suicide, Durkheim (1951) argued that married persons' greater emotional well-being (measured by their relatively lower rates of suicide) is due to their greater social integration in society. Influenced by Durkheim's early insights, sociologists generally believe that similar to other adult social relationships, marriage connects individuals to a broad array of people, which is essential for the development and maintenance of emotional well-being in adulthood (House et al. 1988). Empirical research is, however, inconsistent about marital status differences in social integration; for example, Putnam (2000) and Gerstel and Sarkisan (2006) find that marriage is a "greedy" institution, and that the married report less rather than more engagement in the community than their non-married peers. At the same time, other studies indicate that one of the reasons why divorce and widowhood have deleterious mental health consequences is because they disrupt individuals' social networks (Gerstel et al. 1985; Umberson et al. 1992). It is likely that these inconsistent findings are due to the different ways social integration is conceptualized and measured across studies. While the married are not more involved in the larger community than the non-married, they are more likely than the non-married to have an intimate partner they could confide in and from whom they receive emotional, instrumental (or practical), and financial support (Turner and Turner 1999).

In the 1980s, Kessler and Essex (1982) argued that the married enjoy greater emotional well-being than the non-married because they have more psychosocial resources (i.e., greater social support, mastery and self-esteem), which not only improve mental health but also render them more resilient than the non-married to the negative emotional effects of acute and chronic stress. Drawing on insights from symbolic interaction, Thoits (1986) argued that marriage also provides individuals with a sense of purpose and meaning in life and an important social identity, which have positive effects on mental health as well as buffer the negative emotional impact of life stress. Indeed, studies show that in addition to reporting higher levels of emotional well-being, the married are less vulnerable than the non-married to undesirable life events (Kessler and Essex 1982; Thoits 1986) and chronic strains (Pearlin and Johnson 1977; Simon 1998). Though not yet explored, it is possible that in addition to their greater social support, psychosocial resources and sense of purpose in life, the married experience lower levels of distress and vulnerability because they feel that they *matter* to others—particularly their spouse. Of course, the married also tend to have greater financial resources than the non-married—a pivotal factor that helps explain why single-parents, especially those headed by women, are among the most stressed and distressed social groups in the U.S. (Avison et al. 2007; Carr and Springer 2010; McLanahan 1983; Pearlin and Johnson 1977).

2.2.2.3 Variations in Mental Health Among Married and Non-married Adults

While much of the earlier research focused on documenting marital status differences in distress and vulnerability, studies over the past two decades tend to focus on identifying the social conditions under which marriage is more or less emotionally beneficial; not surprisingly, this research shows that the mental health advantage of marriage is greater for men and women in more than less equitable marriages (Lennon and Rosenfield 1995; Lively et al. 2010; Ross et al. 1983) as well as in higher than lower quality marriages (Hawkins and Booth 2005; Umberson et al. 1996; Williams 2003). In a highly innovative study, Wheaton (1990) found that under certain conditions (i.e., a high level of prior on-going stress), divorce and widowhood actually improve mental health; Wheaton argues that for this group of people, divorce and widowhood represent "stress relief." In view of these findings, it is possible that non-married adults are less distressed than persons in highly stressful marriages; persons who are "single by choice" may also enjoy the same high level of emotional well-being as their married counterparts. Since they are a growing population (Klinenberg 2012), it is important for future research on marriage and mental health to assess whether this is the case.

There is some indirect evidence that persons who choose to be single are not more distressed than their married peers; Simon and Marcussen (Simon and Marcussen 1999) found that persons who hold strong beliefs about the importance of marriage derive a greater mental health benefit from the transition to marriage and remarriage than persons who do not hold strong pro-marriage beliefs. On the flip side, the negative impact of divorce is greater for persons who attach more than less importance to marriage. Although we focused on beliefs about the importance of marriage as moderators of the marital status-mental health association, pro-marriage beliefs may help explain why the marital status gap in mental health is greater between currently and formerly than between currently and never-married persons (Umberson and Williams 1999).

In addition to documenting variation in emotional well-being among the married that is due to variation in marital equity, marital quality, marital stress and marital beliefs, sociologists have been examining heterogeneity in the mental health of non-married adults. In response to increases in non-marital heterosexual cohabitation over the past several decades, researchers have investigated the extent to which these marriage-like relationships offer the same mental health benefit as conventional marriage. Marcussen (2005) finds that men and women in non-marital cohabiting relationships report significantly more depressive symptoms and substance problems than married persons, which is partially explained by their poorer quality relationships (see Brown 2000 for similar results). In her study of social attachments and mental health, Ross (1995) shows that while persons in cohabiting relationships report more depressive symptoms than the married, they enjoy better mental health than single adults. Unfortunately, Ross did not compare the mental health of romantically involved persons who are not co-residing with their partner to persons living with their romantic partner as well as non-romantically involved adults. In a study that focused on emerging adults, Barrett and I (Simon and Barrett 2010) found that young men and women in a romantic relationship report fewer symptoms of depression and substance problems than their non-romantically involved peers. Recent trends in marriage—including the delay of first marriage, non-marital childbearing and increasing rates of non-marital heterosexual cohabitation—as well as cultural shifts undergirding these changes in marital patterns in the U.S. among current cohorts of young adults may narrow the marital status gap in mental health in the next decades of the 21st century. Potentially foreshadowing these trends, a very recent study (Uecker 2012) indicates that married young adults exhibit levels of distress that are similar to those of young adults in any kind of romantic relationship.

Although we have a great deal more to learn about the mental health of the increasingly diverse population of unmarried adults, research is clear about the mental health of single-parents who, due to a number of social and cultural factors, are disproportionately women. Studies consistently document that single-mothers living with dependent children report significantly more depressive symptoms than their married counterparts (Avison et al. 2007; Evenson and Simon 2005; McLanahan 1983; Pearlin and Johnson 1977; Simon 1998). Single-mothers greater distress is due in large part to their greater exposure and vulnerability to a variety of chronic stressors, including the stress of combining work and family responsibilities as well as financial stress (Avison et al. 2007; Pearlin and Johnson 1977; Simon 1998). In fact, social scientists argue that the persistence of the gender gap in earnings, coupled with the increase in female-headed single-parent households, are responsible for the feminization of poverty—a mounting social problem in the U.S. (Christopher et al. 2002; McLanahan and Kelly 2006). Single-mothers' higher levels of emotional distress, especially among those who are poor, have consequences for children's mental health. Studies show that there is an intergenerational transmission of emotional distress and that children growing up in poor single-parent families are significantly more likely to have internalizing and externalizing mental health problems in childhood, adolescence, and young adulthood than children who grew up in two-parent families and female-headed single-parent families that are not poor (Amato and Cheadle 2005; McLeod and Shanahan 1993, 1996).

At the same time that research is clear about the mental health of single-mothers and their children, we know far less about the emotional well-being of both custodial and non-custodial single-fathers as well as non-custodial mothers. Because they continue to be perceived by self and others as "deviant," non-custodial mothers may be even more distressed than single-mothers. In support of this idea, Evenson and I (2005) found that non-custodial mothers of young children report significantly more depressive symptoms than single-mothers residing with their minor offspring. Moreover, despite the preponderance of depression among women, we found that non-custodial fathers actually report significantly more depressive symptoms than custodial single-mothers and fathers residing with their young children. We attributed these findings to non-custodial fathers' lack of involvement in their children's everyday lives, which is highly stressful. Given the recent increase in non-martial childbearing among highly educated women (Cherlin 2010), researchers should compare their level of stress and emotional well-being relative to their less educated and affluent counterparts. Although studies show that parents are more distressed than non-parents (Evenson and Simon 2005), this particular group of single-mothers may enjoy higher levels of well-being than their less educated and solvent peers; they may also enjoy better mental health than working mothers in non-equitable marital relationships.

2.2.2.4 What Have We Learned About Marital Status and Mental Health Over the Past Two Decades?

In sum, sociological research over the past decades consistently documents that marriage confers a number of psychological benefits to men and women, which contribute to their higher levels of emotional well-being. Although they are not necessarily more socially integrated than the non-married, the married do report more social support and both psychosocial and financial resources that improve mental health as well as protect them from negative effects of life stress. At the same time, studies over the past 20 years reveals considerable heterogeneity in mental health among the married that reflects variations in marital equity, marital quality, marital stress and marital beliefs; recent research also documents considerable heterogeneity in mental health among the increasing diverse population of non-married adults—which includes both formerly and never-married adults who have and do not have dependent children, single-parents residing with dependent offspring, non-custodial parents of young children, persons in a variety of non-marital intimate relationships as well as adults who are single-by-choice. The take away message from this body of work is that intimate social relationships—including but not limited to—marital relationships, are associated with improved mental health among women and men.

However, while this body of work has undoubtedly increased our understanding of an array of social factors underlying the relationship between marital status and mental health, there are nonetheless several important gaps in knowledge about the link between intimate social relationships and emotional well-being. Once again, due to space limitations I will only comment on a couple of gaps that I think are most critical for future research to address.

2.2.2.5 Some Current Gaps in Knowledge About Intimate Relationships and Mental Health

In addition to the need for more research on age, race, ethnic, and socioeconomic status variations in the marital status-mental health association among women and among men, we need more research on the ways in which recent social changes in marriage and marriage-like relationships affect individuals' emotional well-being.

A question based on very recent social change that begs for more theoretical and empirical attention is whether men and women in same-sex intimate relationships (including non-marital cohabiting as well as state-sanctioned marital relationships) enjoy the same mental health benefit as their heterosexual peers. At the time this chapter was written, 13 states have extended legal marriage rights to gays and lesbians, which provides a unique opportunity for researchers to compare the emotional well-being of men and women in heterosexual and homosexual marriage (as well as men and women in hetero- and same-sex non-marital cohabiting relationships). Umberson (2012) is taking the lead on this important and theoretically rich topic and has recently collected data on these different types of partnered women and men. Although only time will tell, I strongly suspect that the mental health advantage of marriage is as great, if not greater, for persons in same-sex than in heterosexual relationships because they have fought so long and hard for this privilege. Borrowing Wheaton's concept that I discussed above (Wheaton 1990), the transition to marriage may represent "stress relief" for married gay and lesbian persons who had been denied this civil right relative to their heterosexual peers. At the same time, researchers should also assess the mental health of the LBGTQ community in states that are openly hostile to sexual minorities—particularly in states that have constitutional bans on same-sex marriage and adoption. Recent theory and research on the mental health consequences of perceived stigma and discrimination (Link and Phelan 1999) would provide a useful model for such research.

We also need more prospective studies on the mental health of current cohorts of young adults who, due to a confluence of broad social, economic and cultural forces, are transitioning to adulthood in a context that is different than the context in which their parents came of age. Sociologists note that the transition to adulthood is now a more prolonged period in the life course than it was in the past (Furstenberg et al. 2004). Given the need for more training and education to be competitive in an economy that provides limited employment opportunities for young people, current cohorts of young adults are postponing marriage until their late twenties. At the same time, young women are obtaining higher levels of education than young men, while rates of unemployment are higher for males than females (Kimmel 2009). These social changes, along with the upsurge in non-marital childbearing, are altering the meaning of marriage for young men and women in ways that are not currently well understood; although we do not yet know what their marriages will look like, we do know that marriage is no longer a marker of adulthood and the period of experimentation with non-marital intimate relationships is occupying a longer period of young adults' life course. What these social changes portend for men's and women's mental health before and once they marry is still unclear but it is likely that their marriages will be different from those of their parents. These and other recent social changes in gender and marriage will require sociologists of mental health to rethink some of their assumptions about the emotional advantage of marriage and disadvantage of unmarried statuses in the 21st century. Rather than continuing to focus on marital status differences in emotional well-being, changing marriage patterns in the U.S. behoove researchers to examine the mental health of adults who are and are not in an intimate social relationship—including those who are legally married, those in a committed marriage-like relationship and those not residing with their romantic partner. The marital status gap in mental health may be narrower for current than previous cohorts of adults as new forms of non-marital intimate relationships become the norm.

2.3 Conclusions

As I noted at the beginning of this chapter, the past two decades of sociological research on mental health has made significant theoretical, analytical and substantive progress in our understanding of *how* and *why* people's gender and marital status influence their emotional well-being. Building on but also going beyond theory and research from the 1970s and 1980s when scholarship on the relationships between gender, marital status and mental health first gained momentum, the last 20 years of scholarship has increased our knowledge about social structural, social psychological and sociocultural factors that contribute to persistent gender and marital status differences in emotional well-being. In light of profound social changes in gender and social relationships that have been evolving in the U.S. over the past several decades, I attempted to take stock of the state of current knowledge about the impact of social roles and intimate (including, but not limited to, marital) relationships on men's and women's emotional well-being. Overall, the large body of work on this topic indicates that although some social changes have created greater opportunities for men and women and are associated with increased emotional well-being, others are highly stressful and detrimental for their mental health.

The stress process framework, which first appeared in the late 1970s and early 1980s (Pearlin 1989; Pearlin and Lieberman 1979; Pearlin and Schooler 1978), has stood the test of time and continues to be a dominant explanation of observed gender and marital status differences in emotional well-being during this period of rapid social change. At the same time, researchers have been paying close attention to the larger social, economic and cultural context in which men and women's lives are embedded, the proximate social conditions under which their social roles and relationships are emotionally beneficial or harmful for them as well as the different ways they express mental health problems. By identifying macro- and meso-level social causes of micro-level emotional processes, this new wave of research on gender and marital status disparities in mental health exemplifies the power of the sociological perspective.

With regard to gender inequality in mental health, this research indicates that despite women's increasingly expansive roles in the workplace and family, they continue to report more depressive symptoms than men. The higher rate of depression among women in the U.S. is partially due to persistent gender inequalities in the workplace and family—including the relatively lower wages they receive for the work they do outside the home, the inequitable division of labor within the home, their perceived lack of control over life circumstances as well as their continued responsibility for providing primary care to others while holding a job. Indeed, it appears that current cohorts of employed women are struggling to reconcile their responsibilities and identities as paid workers and mothers.

However, the inclusion of multiple dimensions of mental health in recent studies—particularly male and female typical mental health problems—provides new insight into men's sources of emotional distress and vulnerability. In my view, one of the most important findings from sociological research on mental health over the past two decades is that males and females express emotional upset in different ways and that women are neither more distressed nor more vulnerable than men in general. Indeed, it appears that stressors associated with caregiving tend to be more distressing for women, while stressors involving breadwinning tend to be more distressing for men—at least among the married. Still other stressful life experiences (e.g., divorce and widowhood) are equally distressing for women and men. Thus, rather than continuing to focus exclusively on the social determinants of depression among women, these nuanced gendered patterns behoove sociologists to continue identifying which stressors that are more distressing for women, which are more distressing for men, and which are equally distressing for women and men. The findings of this research are important in their own right but also provide insight into relative importance of work and family identities for women and men.

A critical issue going forward is whether these gendered patterns of distress and vulnerability vary by race, ethnicity, socioeconomic status, age, sexual orientation and LBGTQ identity. Our understanding of the significance of gender for mental health will be greatly enhanced when we focus on the intersection of gender with these other social statuses as well as the interplay between social and biological factors that may contribute to gender differences in the expression of emotional upset. The observation that gender differences in rates of internalizing and externalizing mental health problems first emerge in adolescence require sociologists to look beyond the structure, nature and meaning of men's and women's adult social roles for keys to the complex relationship between gender and mental health.

With regard to the relationship between marital status and mental health, the past two decades of scholarship indicate that for current cohorts of adults, marriage—particularly high quality, low stress and equitable marriage—continues to be associated with higher levels of well-being. In addition to having more financial and psychosocial resources and social support, the married may have a greater sense of purpose and meaning in life than the non-married, which improve mental health and buffer the negative emotional effects of life stress. One of the most important findings from this research is that the advantages of marriage and remarriage, and disadvantages of unmarried statuses, are evident among both women and men and reflect both social causation and selection processes. At the same time, this research also reveals that while they do not confer the same emotional advantage as marriage among current cohorts of adults, persons in non-marital intimate relationships (including but not limited to cohabiting relationships) enjoy better mental health than persons who do not have an intimate partner.

Indeed, social changes in marital patterns that were nascent at the close of the twentieth century—including increases in heterosexual and same-sex marriage-like relationships, same-sex marriage, female headed single-parent households as well as persons who are single-by-choice—are creating greater heterogeneity in the population of unmarried adults in the U.S. today; increasing heterogeneity among the non-married requires sociologists of mental health to go beyond simple comparisons of the emotional well-being of married and non-married adults—particularly as the next cohorts of men and women transition to adulthood. Armed with more nuanced theories, sophisticated data analytic techniques and recent panel data, sociologists of mental health are in an excellent position to track the continued significance of gender and social (including marital) relationships for mental health in the early decades of the 21st century as new cohorts of men and women come of age and as our population becomes increasingly diverse.

Acknowledgments I am grateful to Robert Johnson, Bruce Link, and Jay Turner for inviting my contribution to this volume. I also thank the two anonymous reviewers for their excellent suggestions as well as Debra Umberson and Mieke Beth Thomeer for providing abstracts of all articles published over the past two decades in the *Journal of Health and Social Behavior* on the topics of gender, marital status, and mental health.

References

Amato, P. R., & Cheadle, J. (2005). The long reach of divorce: divorce and child-well-being across three generations. *Journal of Marriage and Family, 67*, 191–206.
Aneshensel, C. S. (1992). Social stress: Theory and research. *Annual Review of Sociology, 18*, 15–38.
Aneshensel, C. S., Frerichs, R. R., & Clark, V. A. (1981). Family roles and sex differences in depression. *Journal of Health and Social Behavior, 22*, 379–393.
Aneshensel, C. S., Rutter, C. M., & Lachenbruch, P. A. (1991). Social structure, stress, and mental health: Competing conceptual and analytic models. *American Sociological Review, 56*, 166–178.
Avison, W., Ali, J., & Walters, D. (2007). Family structure, stress, and psychological distress: A demonstration of the impact of differential exposure. *Journal of Health and Social Behavior, 62*, 911–926.
Avison, W., & McAlpine, D. (1992). Gender differences in symptoms of depression among adolescents. *Journal of Health and Social Behavior, 33*, 77–96.
Barrett, A. E. (2000). Marital trajectories and mental health. *Journal of Health and Social Behavior, 41*, 451–464.
Barrett, A. E. (2005). Gendered experiences in midlife: Implications for age identity. *Journal of Aging Studies, 19*, 163–183.
Bernard, J. (1982). *The future of marriage*. New Haven: Yale University.
Bianchi, S. M., & Milke, M. A. (2010). Work and family research in the first decade of the 21st century. *Journal of Marriage and the Family, 72*, 705–725.
Bianchi, S. M., Robinson, J. P., & Milke, M. A. (2007). *Changing rhythms of American family life*. New York: Russell Sage.
Bird, C. E. (1999). Gender, household labor, and psychological distress: The impact of the amount and division of housework. *Journal of Health and Social Behavior, 40*, 32–45.
Bird, C. E., & Rieker, P. P. (1999). Gender matters: An integrated model for understanding men's and women's health. *Social Science and Medicine, 48*, 745–755.

Bird, C. E., & Rieker, P. P. (2008). *Gender and health: The effects of constrained choices and social policies*. New York: Cambridge University Press.

Booth, A., & Amato, P. (1991). Divorce and psychological stress. *Journal of Health and Social Behavior, 32*, 396–407.

Brown, S. (2000). The effect of union type on psychological well-being: Depression among cohabitors versus marrieds. *Journal of Health and Social Behavior, 41*, 241–255.

Caputo, J., & Simon, R. W. (2013). Physical limitations and emotional well-being: Gender and marital status variations. *Journal of Health and Social Behavior, 54*, 241–257.

Carr, D., & Springer, K. W. (2010). Advances in families and health research in the 21st century. *Journal of Marriage and the Family, 72*, 744–761.

Cherlin, A. (2010). Demographic trends in the United States: A review of research in the 2000s. *Journal of Marriage and the Family, 72*, 403–419.

Christopher, K., England, P., Smeeding, T. M., & Phillips, K. R. (2002). Nations: Single motherhood, the market, and the state. *Sociological Perspectives, 45*, 219–242.

Cleary, P. D., & Mechanic, D. (1983). Sex differences in psychological distress among married people. *Journal of Health and Social Behavior, 24*, 111–121.

Conger, R. D., Lorenz, F. O., Elder, G. H, Jr, Simons, R. L., & Ge, X. (1993). Husband and wife differences in response to undesirable life events. *Journal of Health and Social Behavior, 34*, 71–88.

Dohrenwend, B. S., & Dohrenwend, B. S. (1977). Sex differences in psychiatric disorders. *American Journal of Sociology, 81*, 1447–1454.

Durkheim, E. (1951). *Suicide: A study in sociology*. New York: Free Press.

Ensminger, M. E., & Celantano, D. D. (1990). Gender differences in the effect of unemployment on psychological distress. *Social Science and Medicine, 30*, 469–477.

Evenson, R., & Simon, R. W. (2005). Clarifying the relationship between parenthood and depression. *Journal of Health and Social Behavior, 46*, 358–3411.

Fausto-Sterling, A. (1992). *Biological theories about women and men*. New York: Basic Books.

Forthofer, M. S., Kessler, R. C., Story, A. L., & Gotlib, I. H. (1996). The effects of psychiatric disorders on the probability and timing of first marriage. *Journal of Health and Social Behavior, 37*, 121–132.

Frank Jr, F., Kennedy, S., McLoyd, V. C., Rumbaut, R. G., & Settersten Jr, R. A. (2004). Growing up is harder to do. *Contexts* 3: 33–41.

Gerson, K. (2011). *The unfinished revolution: Coming of age in a new era of gender, work, and family*. New York: Oxford.

Gerstel, N., Riessman, C. K., & Rosenfield, S. (1985). Explaining the symptomology of separated and divorced women and men: The role of material conditions and social networks. *Social Forces, 64*, 84–101.

Gerstel, N., & Sarkisian, N. (2006). Marriage: the good, the bad, and the ugly. *Contexts, 5*, 16–21.

Glass, J., & Fujimoto, T. (1994). Housework, paid work, and depression among husbands and wives. *Journal of Health and Social Behavior, 35*, 179–191.

Gore, S., Aseltine, R., & Cotton, S. (1992). Social structure, life stress, and depressive symptoms in a high-school-age population. *Journal of Health and Social Behavior, 33*, 97–113.

Gore, S., & Mangione, T. (1983). Social roles, sex roles, and psychological distress: Additive and interactive models. *Journal of Health and Social Behavior, 24*, 300–312.

Gove, W. R. (1972). The Relationship between Sex Roles, Marital Status and Mental Illness. *Social Forces, 51*, 34–44.

Gove, W., & Tudor, J. F. (1973). Adult sex roles and mental illness. *American Journal of Sociology, 78*, 50–73.

Hagan, J., & Foster, H. (2003). S/He's a Rebel: Toward a sequential theory of delinquency and gendered pathways to disadvantage in emerging adulthood. *Social Forces, 82*, 53–86.

Hawkins, D., & Booth, A. (2005). Unhappily ever after: Effects of long-term, low- quality marriages on well-being. *Social Forces, 84*, 451–471.

Hill, S. A., & Sprague, J. (1999). Parenting in black and white families: The interaction of gender with race and class. *Gender and Society, 13*, 480–502.
Hochschild, A. R. (1979). Emotion work, feeling rules, and social structure. *American Journal of Sociology, 85*, 551–575.
Hochschild, A. R. (1983). *The managed heart: Notes on the commercialization of human feeling.* Berkeley: University of California.
Hochschild, A. (1989). *The second shift: Working parents and the revolution at home.* New York: Viking.
Hopcroft, R. L., & Bradley, D. B. (2007). The sex difference in depression across 29 countries. *Social Forces, 85*, 1483–1507.
Horwitz, A. V., White, H. R., & Howell-White, S. (1996). The use of multiple outcomes in stress research: A case study of gender differences in responses to marital dissolution. *Journal of Health and Social Behavior, 37*, 278–291.
House, J. S., Landis, K., & Umberson, D. (1988). Social relationships and health. *Science, 241*, 540–545.
Kessler, R. C. (1979a). Stress, social status, and psychological distress. *Journal of Health and Social Behavior, 20*, 259–272.
Kessler, R. C. (1979b). A strategy for studying differential vulnerability to the psychological consequences of stress. *Journal of Health and Social Behavior, 20*, 100–108.
Kessler, R. C. (2003). Epidemiology of women and depression. *Journal of Affective Disorders, 74*, 5–13.
Kessler, R. C., & Essex, M. (1982). Marital status and depression: The importance of coping resources. *Social Forces, 6*, 484–507.
Kessler, R. C., & Jr, J. M. (1982). The effect of wives' employment on the mental health of married men and women. *American Sociological Review, 47*, 216–227.
Kessler, R. C., McGonagle, K. A., Schwartz, M., Blazer, D. G., & Nelson, C. B. (1993). Sex and depression in the national comorbidity survey I: Lifetime prevalence, chronicity, and recurrence. *Journal of Affective Disorders, 25*, 85–96.
Kessler, R. C., McGonagle, K. A., Zhao, S., Nelson, C. B., Hughes, M., Eshleman, S., et al. (1994). Lifetime and 12-month prevalence of DSM-III R psychiatric disorders in the United States: Results from the national comorbidity survey. *Archives of General Psychiatry, 51*, 8–19.
Kessler, R. C., & McLeod, J. D. (1984). Sex differences in vulnerability to undesirable life events. *American Sociological Review, 49*, 620–631.
Kessler, R. C., & McRae, J. A. (1984). Trends in the relationships of sex and marital status to psychological distress. *Research in Community and Mental Health, 4*, 109–130.
Kimmel, M. (2009). *Guyland: The perilous world of where boys become men.* New York: Harper.
Klinenberg, E. (2012). *Going solo: The extraordinary rise and surprising appeal of living alone.* New York: Penguin.
Ladner, J. (1995). *Tomorrow's tomorrow: The black woman.* Lincoln: University of Nebraska Press.
Lennon, M. C. (1987). Sex differences in distress: The impact of gender and work roles. *Journal of Health and Social Behavior, 28*, 290–305.
Lennon, M. C., & Rosenfield, S. (1995). Relative fairness and the division of household work. *American Journal of Sociology, 100*, 506–531.
Link, B. G., & Phelan, J. C. (1999). Labeling and stigma. In C. S. Aneshensel & J. C. Phelan (Eds.), *Handbook of the sociology of mental health* (pp. 481–493). New York: Kluwer.
Lively, K., Steelman, L. C., & Powell, B. (2010). Equity, emotion, and household division of labor. *Social Psychology Quarterly, 73*, 358–379.
Mabry, J. B., & Kiecolt, Jill. (2005). Anger in black and white: race, alienation, and anger. *Journal of Health and Social Behavior, 46*, 85–101.
Marcussen, K. (2005). Explaining differences in mental health between married and cohabiting individuals. *Social Psychology Quarterly, 68*, 239–257.

Marks, N. F., & Lambert, J. D. (1998). Marital status continuity and change among young and midlife adults: Longitudinal effects on psychological well-being. *Journal of Family Issues, 19*, 652–686.

Mastekaasa, Arne. (1992). Marriage and psychological well-being: some evidence on selection into marriage. *Journal of Marriage and the Family, 54*, 901–911.

McLanahan, S. (1983). Family structure and stress: A longitudinal comparison of two-parent and female-headed families. *Journal of Marriage and the Family, 45*, 347–357.

McLanahan, S., & Kelly, E. (2006). The feminization of poverty: Past and future. In J. Chafetz (Ed.), *Handbook of the sociology of gender* (pp. 127–145). New York: Plenum.

McLeod, J. D., & Shanahan, M. J. (1993). Poverty, parenting, and children's mental health. *American Sociological Review, 58*, 351–366.

McLeod, J. D., & Shanahan, M. J. (1996). Trajectories of poverty and children's mental health. *Journal of Health and Social Behavior, 37*, 207–220.

McMullin, J. A., & Cairney, J. (2004). Self-esteem and the intersection of age, class, and gender. *Journal of Aging Studies, 18*, 75–90.

Menaghan, E. G. (1985). Depressive affect and subsequent divorce. *Journal of Family Issues, 6*, 296–306.

Menaghan, E. G. (1989). Role changes and psychological well-being: Variations in effects by gender and role repertoire. *Social Forces, 3*, 693–714.

Meyers, J. K., Weissman, M. M., Tischler, G. L., Holzer, C. E., Leaf, P. J., Orvaschel, H., et al. (1984). Six-month prevalence of psychiatric disorders in three communities. *Archives of General Psychiatry, 41*, 959–967.

Miller, S. M., & Kirsh, N. (1989). Sex differences in cognitive coping with stress. In R. C. Barnette, L. Biener, & G. K. Baruch (Eds.), *Gender and stress* (pp. 278–307). New York: Aldine de Gruyter.

Mirowsky, J. (1996). Age and the gender gap in depression. *Journal of Health and Social Behavior, 37*, 362–380.

Mirowsky, J., & Ross, C. (2006). *Social causes of psychological distress*. New York: Aldine.

Needham, B., & Hill, T. (2010). Do gender differences in mental health contribute to gender differences in physical health? *Social Science and Medicine, 71*, 1472–1479.

Newman, J. P. (1986). Gender, life strains, and depression. *Journal of Health and Social Behavior, 27*, 161–178.

Nomaguchi, K., Milke, M., & Bianchi, S. (2005). Time strains and psychological well-being: Do dual earner mothers and fathers differ? *Journal of Family Issues, 26*, 756–792.

Offer, S., & Schneider, B. (2011). Revisiting the gender gap in time-use patterns: Multitasking and well-being among mothers and fathers in dual-earner families. *American Sociological Review, 76*, 809–833.

Parsons, Talcott. (1955). *Family socialization and interaction processes*. Glencoe: Free Press.

Pearlin, L. I. (1975). Sex roles and depression. In N. Datan & L. Ginsberg (Eds.), *Proceedings of the fourth lifespan developmental psychology conference: Normative life crises* (pp. 191–208). New York: Academic Press.

Pearlin, L. I. (1989). The sociological study of stress. *Journal of Health and Social Behavior, 30*, 241–256.

Pearlin, L. I., & Johnson, J. (1977). Marital status, life strains, and depression. *American Sociological Review, 42*, 704–715.

Pearlin, L. I., & Lieberman, M. A. (1979). Social sources of emotional distress. In R. Simmons (Ed.), *Research and community mental health* (Vol. 1, pp. 217–248). New York: JAI Press.

Pearlin, L. I., & Schooler, C. (1978). The structure of coping. *Journal of Health and Social Behavior, 19*, 2–21.

Pescosolido, B. A., Perry, B. L., Scott Long, J., & Martin, J. K. (2008). Under the influence of genetics: How trans-disciplinary leads us to rethink social pathways to illness. *American Journal of Sociology, 114*(Supplement), S171–S201.

Powell, B., Bolzendahl, C., Geist, C., & Steelman, L. C. (2010). *Same sex relations and Americans' definition of family*. New York: Russell Sage.

Putnam, R. D. (2000). *Bowling alone*. New York: Simon and Schuster.
Ridgeway, C. (2011). *Framed by gender: How gender inequality persists in the modern world*. New York: Oxford University Press.
Rieker, P. P., & Bird, C. E. (2008). Rethinking gender differences in health: Why we need to integrate social and biological perspectives. *The Journals of Gerontology, Series B, 60*(2), S40–S47.
Robins, L. N., & Regier, D. A. (Eds.). (1994). *Psychiatric disorders in America: The epidemiologic catchment area study*. New York: Free Press.
Robins, R. W., & Trzesniewski, K. H. (2005). Self-esteem development across the lifespan. *Current Directions in Psychological Science, 14*, 158–162.
Rosenfield, S. (1980). Sex differences in depression: Do women always have higher rates? *Journal of Health and Social Behavior, 21*, 33–42.
Rosenfield, S. (1989). The effects of women's employment: Personal control and sex differences in mental health. *Journal of Health and Social Behavior, 30*, 77–91.
Rosenfield, S. (1992). The costs of sharing: Wives' employment and husbands' mental health. *Journal of Health and Social Behavior, 33*, 213–225.
Rosenfield, S. (1999a). Gender and mental health: Do women have more psychopathology, men more, or both the same (and why)? In A. V. Horwitz, & T. L. Scheid (Eds.), *Handbook for the study of mental health: Social contexts, theories, and systems* (pp. 349–360). Cambridge: Cambridge Press.
Rosenfield, S. (1999b). Splitting the difference: gender, the self, and mental health. In C. S. Aneshensel, & J. C. Phelan (Eds.), *Handbook of the sociology of mental health* (pp. 209–224). New York: Kluwer Academic/Plenum Publishers.
Rosenfield, S. (2012). Triple jeopardy? Mental health at the intersection of gender, race, and class. *Social Science and Medicine, 74*, 1791–1801.
Rosenfield, S., Lennon, M. C., & White, H. R. (2005). The self and mental health: Self-salience and the emergence of internalizing and externalizing problems. *Journal of Health and Social Behavior, 46*, 323–340.
Rosenfield, S., & Mouzon, D. (2013). Gender and mental health. In C. S. Aneshensel, J. C. Phelan, & A. Bierman (Eds.), *Handbook of the sociology of mental health* (2nd ed., pp. 277–298), New York: Kluwer.
Rosenfield, S., Philips, J., & White, H. (2006). Gender, race and the self in mental health and crime. *Social Problems, 53*, 161–185.
Rosenfield, S., Vertefuille, J., & McAlpine, D. (2000). Gender stratification and mental health: dimensions of the self. *Social Psychology Quarterly, 63*, 208–223.
Ross, C. (1995). Re-conceptualizing marital status as a continuum of social attachment. *Journal of Marriage and the Family, 57*, 129–140.
Ross, C., & Mirowsky, J. (1988). Childcare and emotional adjustment to wives' employment. *Journal of Health and Social Behavior, 29*, 127–138.
Ross, C., Mirowsky, J., & Huber, J. (1983). Dividing work, sharing work, and in-between: Marriage patters and depression. *American Sociological Review, 48*, 809–823.
Ross, C., & Van Willigen, M. (1996). Gender, parenthood, and anger. *Journal of Marriage and the Family, 58*, 572–584.
Roxburgh, S. (1996). Gender differences in work and well-being: Effects of exposure and vulnerability. *Journal of Health and Social Behavior, 37*, 265–277.
Schnittker, J. (2008). Happiness and success: genes, families, and the psychological effects of socioeconomic position and social support. *American Journal of Sociology, 114*(Supplement), S233–S259.
Simon, R. W. (1992). Parental role strains, salience of parental identity, and gender differences in psychological distress. *Journal of Health and Social Behavior, 33*, 25–35.
Simon, R. W. (1995). Gender, multiple roles, role meaning, and mental health. *Journal of Health and Social Behavior, 36*, 182–194.
Simon, R. W. (1997). The meanings individuals attach to role identities and their implications for mental health. *Journal of Health and Social Behavior, 38*, 256–274.

Simon, R. W. (1998). Assessing sex differences in vulnerability among employed parents: The importance of marital status. *Journal of Health and Social Behavior, 39*, 37–53.

Simon, R. W. (2000). The importance of culture in sociological theory and research on stress and mental health: A missing link? In C. Bird, P. Conrad, & A. Fremont (Eds.), *Handbook of medical sociology* (5th ed., pp. 68–78). New York: Prentice Hall.

Simon, R. W. (2002). Revisiting the relationships among gender, marital status, and mental health. *American Journal of Sociology, 107*, 1065–1096.

Simon, R. W. (2007). Contributions of the sociology of mental health for understanding the social antecedents, social regulation, and social distribution of emotion. In W. Avison, J. McLeod, & B. Pescosilido (Eds.), *Mental Health, Social mirror* (pp. 239–274). New York: Springer.

Simon, R. W., & Barrett, A. E. (2010). Non-marital romantic relationships and mental health in early adulthood: Does the association differ for women and men?. *Journal of Health and Social Behavior, 51*, 168–182.

Simon, R. W., & Lively, K. (2010). Sex, anger, and depression. *Social Forces, 88*, 1543–1568.

Simon, R. W., & Marcussen, K. (1999). Marital transitions, marital beliefs, and mental health. *Journal of Health and Social Behavior, 40*, 111–125.

Simon, R. W., & Nath, Leda K. (2004). Gender and emotion in the U.S.: Do men and women differ in self-reports of feelings and expressive behavior? *American Journal of Sociology, 109*, 1137–1176.

Smith-Lovin, L. (1995). The sociology of affect and emotion. In K. Cook, G. A. Fine, & J. S. House (Eds.), *Sociological perspectives of social psychology* (pp. 118–148). New York: Allyn Bacon.

Springer, K. W., Hankivsky, O., & Bates, L. M. (2012). Gender and health: Relational, intersectional, and biosocial approaches. *Social Science and Medicine, 74*, 1661–1666.

Stevenson, B., & Wolfers, J. (2009). The paradox of declining female happiness. *American Economic Journal: Economic Policy, 1*, 190–225.

Thoits, P. A. (1982). Life stress, social support, and psychological vulnerability: Epidemiological considerations. *Journal of Community Psychology, 10*, 341–362.

Thoits, P. A. (1986). Multiple identities: Examining gender and marital status differences in distress. *American Sociological Review, 51*, 259–272.

Thoits, P. A. (1987). Gender and marital status differences in control and distress: Common stress versus unique stress explanations. *Journal of Health and Social Behavior, 28*, 7–22.

Thoits, P. A. (1989). The sociology of emotions. *Annual Review of Sociology, 15*, 317–342.

Thoits, P. A. (1991). On merging identity theory and stress research. *Social Psychology Quarterly, 54*, 101–112.

Thoits, P. A. (1992). Identity structures and psychological well-being: Gender and marital status comparisons. *Social Psychology Quarterly, 55*, 236–256.

Thoits, P. A. (1995). Stress, coping, and social support: Where are we? What next? *Journal of Health and Social Behavior, 35*(Extra Issue), 53–79.

Thoits, P. A. (2010). Stress and health: Major findings and policy implications. *Journal of Health and Social Behavior, 51*, 41–53.

Turner, R. J., & Roszell P. (1994). Psychosocial resources and the stress process. In W. R. Avison, & I. H. Gotlib (Eds.), *Stress and mental health: Contemporary issues and prospects for the future* (pp. 179–210). New York: Plenum Press.

Turner, R. J., & Avison, W. (1989). Gender and depression: Assessing exposure and vulnerability to life events in a chronically strained population. *Journal of Nervous and Mental Disease, 177*, 443–455.

Turner, R. J., & Marino, F. (1994). Social support and social structure: A descriptive epidemiology. *Journal of Health and Social Behavior, 235*, 193–212.

Turner, R. J., & Turner, J. B. (1999). Social integration and support. In C. S. Aneshensel, & J. C. Phelan (Eds.), *The handbook of the sociology of mental health* (pp. 301–319). New York: Kluwer.

Turner, R. J., Wheaton, B., & Lloyd, D. A. (1995). The epidemiology of social stress. *American Sociological Review, 60*, 104–125.

Uecker, J. E. (2012). Marriage and mental health among young adults. *Journal of Health and Social Behavior, 53*, 67–83.

Ueno, Koji. (2010). Same-Sex experience and mental health during the transition between adolescence and young adulthood. *Sociological Quarterly, 51*, 484–510.

Umberson D. (2012). Marriage, gender and health in lesbian, gay and heterosexual couples. Grant from the Robert Wood Johnson foundation.

Umberson, D., Chen, M. D., House, J. S., Hopkins, K., & Slater, E. (1996). The effect of social relationships on psychological well-being: Are men and women really so different? *American Sociological Review, 61*, 837–857.

Umberson, D., & Kristi, W. (1999). Family status and mental health. In C. S. Aneshensel, & J. C. Phelan (Eds.), *The handbook of the sociology of mental health* (pp. 225–253). New York: Kluwer.

Umberson, D., Wortman, C. A., & Kessler, R. C. (1992). Widowhood and depression: Explaining long-term gender differences in vulnerability. *Journal of Health and Social Behavior, 33*, 10–24.

United States Census Bureau. (2010). Households and families: 2010. 2010 Census briefs. (http://www.census.gov/prod/cen2010/briefs/c2010br-14.pdf).

Wade, T. J., & Pevalin, D. J. (2004). Marital transitions and mental health. *Journal of Health and Social Behavior, 45*, 155–170.

Weissman, M. M., & Klerman, G. L. (1977). Sex differences and the epidemiology of depression. *Archives of General Psychiatry, 34*, 98–111.

Wheaton, B. (1990). Life transitions, role histories, and mental health. *American Sociological Review, 55*, 209–223.

Williams, K. (2003). Has the future of marriage arrived? A contemporary examination of gender, marriage, and psychological well-being. *Journal of Health and Social Behavior, 44*, 470–487.

Williams, D. R., Takeuchi, D., & Adair, R. K. (1992). Marital status and psychiatric disorders among blacks and whites. *Journal of Health and Social Behavior, 33*, 140–157.

World Health Organization. (2000). International consortium of psychiatric epidemiology: Cross-national comparisons of mental disorders. *Bulletin of the World Health Organization, 78*, 413–426.

Yang, Y. (2008). Social inequalities in happiness in the U.S. 1972–2004: An age-period-cohort analysis. *American Sociological Review, 73*, 2004–2026.

Chapter 3
The Stress Process: Its Origins, Evolution, and Future

Carol S. Aneshensel and Uchechi A. Mitchell

Over the past several decades, the Stress Process Model has provided the predominant theoretical foundation for sociological research into the effects of stress on mental health and empirical research continues to substantiate its account of how society shapes the mental health of its members. Its core elements remain as originally formulated by Pearlin et al. (1981) some thirty plus years ago: the influence of the social system on exposure to stressors; parallel effects on access to social and personal resources; and, the role of these resources as mediators and moderators of the effect of stressors on mental health. Wheaton (2010) contends that the Stress Process Model has remained the leading paradigm in sociological stress research at least in part because it is an open system that invites elaboration, extension, and innovation—a potential that has been actualized to a large extent over time. As a result, the Stress Process Model now offers a coherent explanation of why people's chances of having a mental disorder depend upon their location within systems of stratification and their participation in social institutions and relationships—its quintessentially sociological characteristic (Pearlin 1989).[1]

The authors wish to thank Leonard I. Pearlin and an anonymous reviewer for suggestions that enhanced the chapter.

---

[1] There are, of course, other productive sociological approaches to understanding the unequal distribution of mental disorder throughout society. As a case in point, McLeod (2013) attributes mental health disparities partly to social evaluative processes.

C.S. Aneshensel (✉) · U.A. Mitchell
Department of Community Health Sciences, Fielding School of Public Health,
University of California, Los Angeles, CA 90095-1772, USA
e-mail: anshnsl@ucla.edu

U.A. Mitchell
e-mail: uchechi@gmail.com

The ubiquitous use of the word stress in everyday conversation makes the concept both familiar and amorphous because its boundaries seem to include much of daily life. For this reason, it is useful to first define the term stressor, which refers to: (1) the *presence* of environmental threats, challenges, or demands that tax or exceed the individual's ordinary capacity to adapt, and (2) the *absence* of the means to attain sought-after ends (Lazarus 1966; Pearlin 1983; Menaghan 1983; Aneshensel 1992; Wheaton et al. 2013). Stress refers to the arousal of internal physiological responses to the occurrence of a stressor. These responses include activation of key areas of the brain that initiate biological processes designed to protect the organism—fight, flight, or freeze—and to then return the body to homeostasis—an internal state of equilibrium. Key regulatory systems of the body that are involved in this process include the hypothalamic-pituitary-adrenocortical (HPA) axis, the autonomic nervous system and the immune system. Typical psychological responses to stressors include, for example, feeling endangered, besieged, or frustrated. These responses are called distress when they become maladaptive in the form of symptoms of anxiety, depression, and behavioral disorders such as substance abuse (Wheaton et al. 2013). In contrast, the term stressor refers to the external circumstances that challenge or obstruct.

Research on stress and health originated with Selye's (1936) biological model of stress based on laboratory studies with animals using exposure to aversive physical and mental stimuli (e.g., extreme changes in ambient temperature). Selye described the short- and long-term responses to stressors, collectively referred to as the General Adaptation Syndrome and consisting of: (1) an initial stage of alarm and defense, (2) a subsequent stage of resistance or adaptation, and (3) a final stage of exhaustion, the breakdown of physiological systems, or death if exposure persists. Recent research in this tradition focuses on the extent to which constant or repeated exposure to stressors creates structural and functional alterations in systems of the body, such as the cardiovascular and autonomic nervous system and the HPA axis. The cumulative overuse and wearing down of these regulatory systems is referred to as allostatic load (McEwen and Steller 1993) and has been linked to physical and cognitive decline (Karlamangla et al. 2002), symptoms of Post-Traumatic Stress Disorder (Glover 2006), and all-cause mortality (Seeman et al. 2004).

Wheaton (1994; Wheaton et al. 2013) presents an alternative model developed by Smith (1987; cited in Wheaton 1994) as a heuristic device for conceptualizing potential stress responses. "Elastic limit" is a key concept, referring to situations where the level of force exceeds the limits of the structural integrity of a material, leading to strain—its elongation or compression. The material (1) returns to its original shape after the stress is removed if the initial elastic limit is not exceeded, (2) achieves a greater elastic limit by adjusting to elongation or compression up to a finite point, (3) after which it cannot adaptively respond and fractures or breaks down. Wheaton (1994) finds this model useful for conceptualizing responses to stressors because it encompasses the effects of both catastrophic forces (e.g., hurricane-force winds) and continuous forces (e.g., rust), analogous to major life events and chronic stressors—the foci of most sociological stress research (see below). When applied to people, the model implies that coping capacity may increase in response to a stressor, but only until a breaking point is reached. Although this model provides an alternative conceptualization of stress responses, the key ideas of elastic limit, increased coping capacity, and breaking points have yet to be systematically tested.

The propensity to evoke stress inheres within the stressor as the amount of threat or obstruction it would pose on average to most people most of the time, but the extent to which it does elicit a stress response depends upon a number of factors such as the meaning that it is attributed to it or the context in which it occurs. As a result, there typically exists substantial variation among people in responses to the same objective event or circumstance. Some of this variation is idiosyncratic—unique to each individual, and calls for personal explanations as might be sought through introspection.[2] Sociological explanation, in contrast, focuses on the explanation of social patterns in these responses (Pearlin 1989). As a concrete example, women are more affected psychologically than men by boundary-spanning work demands—demands to perform one social role while enacting another role—that lead to a "blurring" of work and family roles (Glavin et al. 2011).

In this paper, we first describe the Stress Process Model as originally formulated by Pearlin et al. (1981). We then chronicle four pivotal points in its evolution, describing their impact as manifest in current research. These developments are: (1) the articulation of the nature of sociological inquiry into stress, (2) the conceptualization and measurement of the stress universe, (3) the debate about psychological distress as a continuum versus discrete disorders as appropriate outcomes for sociological research, and (4) the proposition that multiple outcomes are required to ascertain the mental health consequences of stressors. Given the rich history of innovation in this field, the selection of these developments was a difficult one necessitated by space constraints and it inevitably reflects our own predilections. Several other major advances that contributed to or flowed from these three developments also are identified, including: the differential exposure and differential vulnerability hypotheses, the concept of stress proliferation, and research on the social epidemiology of the stress process. We end with a call for more systematic research into the ways in which the components of the Stress Process Model are related to one another in order to more fully realize its explanatory potential as a system.

3.1 The Stress Process Revisited

In *The Stress Process*, Pearlin et al. (1981) identified a set of core constructs and, most importantly, a system of relationships among these constructs—set within an overarching goal of elaborating the mechanisms through which the organization of

---

[2] Statistically, this unique variation is captured in the error term of regression models, an ironic operationalization of individuality, especially when applied to the very personal experience of mental illness.

society becomes manifest in the mental health of its members. The stated motive was specifying the interconnections among the discrete and disparate findings that were emerging at the time from the rapidly expanding body of research on stress and its health effects.

3.1.1 Conceptualizing the Elements of the Stress Process

The article examined the relationship between life events and chronic stressors, as shown in Fig. 3.1, and in doing so expanded the conceptual boundaries of stressors beyond the contemporary practice of equating stressors with life change events—although it would take quite some time for chronic stressors to gain equal prominence (Wheaton 2010). Life change events were defined at the time as objective occurrences of sufficient magnitude to change the usual activities of most persons or alter their social setting (Rabkin and Streuning 1976; Dohrenwend et al. 1978). Examples are death of a loved one and home foreclosure. The initial conceptualization of any change as stress-provoking soon gave way, however, because undesirable events were found to be most psychologically distressing (Ross and Mirowsky 1979; Thoits 1983). Also, stressors do not necessarily entail change but can be found in the persistence of difficult conditions over time. These chronic stressors typically have a slow and insidious onset, remain problematic over a lengthy time, and have an uncertain ending (Pearlin 1983;

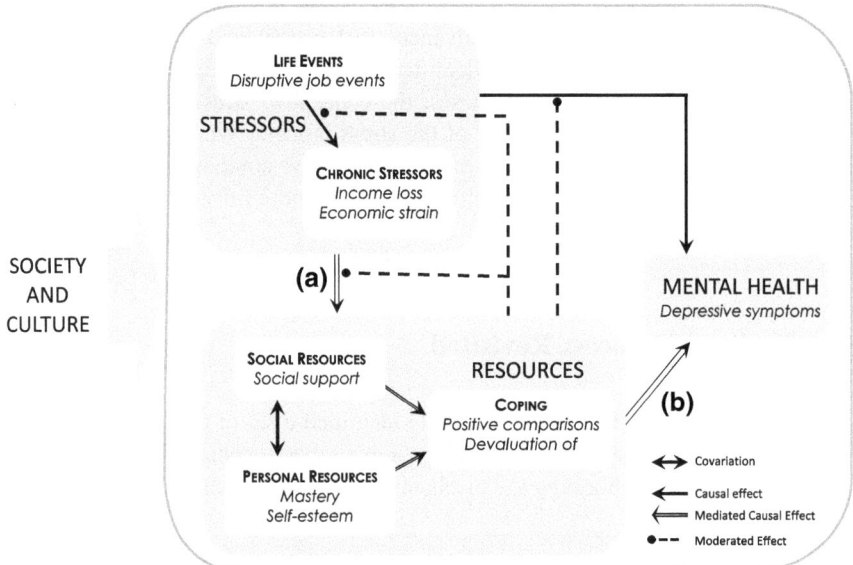

Fig. 3.1 The original stress process model. Based on Pearlin et al. (1981)

Wheaton 1994). Examples include ongoing financial problems and seemingly interminable conflict between spouses.[3]

The Stress Process Model also synthesized emergent concepts in the stress literature pertaining to social and personal resources that may offset the deleterious mental health effects of stressors, honing in on three that were to become mainstays of stress research: social support—the belief that others care about you; and, self-concept in the forms of mastery—the belief that your life-chances are under your own control instead of being determined by fate, chance, or powerful others; and, self-esteem—positive views of oneself. These resources were seen as affecting coping (see Fig. 3.1), which refers to steps people take to avoid or lessen the impact of stressors (Pearlin and Schooler 1978). These actions include: avoiding the stressor in the first place, successfully resolving the stressor when it is unavoidable, managing the meaning of the stressor in ways that reduce its threat; and, keeping adverse emotional reactions within manageable bounds (Pearlin and Aneshensel 1986; Pearlin 1989).

The mental health outcome studied in the original article was depression as indexed by a symptom measure, a choice that foreshadowed the direction followed by the preponderance of subsequent work on the stress process, although major depressive disorder also has figured prominently as an outcome, and as discussed below, these outcomes have been the subject of debate.

3.1.2 A System of Relationships

The Stress Process also presented a system of relationships leading from stress exposure through resources to adverse mental health outcomes, and put the hypothesized system to an empirical test (Pearlin et al. 1981). The investigators posited that the occurrence of life events could lead to the subsequent emergence of chronic stressors, as shown in Fig. 3.1. Making this connection altered the prevailing practices of equating stressors with life change events and conceptualizing life change events as independent occurrences. Analysis of survey data from a sample of Chicago adults substantiated this hypothesis, revealing that disruptive job events, such as involuntary job loss, lowered income and thereby increased economic strain.

In addition, both sources of stress were shown to be depressing to the extent that they diminished the person's self-concept, specifically lessening self-esteem and mastery—thereby incorporating *mediators* into the stress process. Mediation is shown in Fig. 3.1 as the pair of arrows leading (a) from stressors to resources and (b) from resources to mental health outcomes.[4] Equally important, resources

---

[3] However, as Avison and Turner (1988) demonstrated, some events follow the same lengthy time course as chronic stressors so that duration should be measured.

[4] The diminishment of self-concept was conceived of as a mechanism through which life events and chronic strains become stressful, but it has since been considered in the domain of resources, a consequential shift in thinking, as discussed below.

were found to act as *moderators*, weakening the effects of stressors on depressive symptoms. Moderation is shown as the dashed line that intersect a pathway, signifying that it is the pathway that is affected by the moderator, not the constructs that anchor the pathway.[5] Notably, coping and social support also curtailed the effects of disruptive job events at other points in the model, lessening its effects on chronic stressors and mastery. In this way, *The Stress Process* called attention to the interconnections among social and personal factors that influence the impact of stressors on mental health, as distinct from the more common approach of focusing on each factor's distinct contribution to explaining variation in mental health. By tracing indirect effects of stressors on mental health, instead of considering only their main effects, as was the usual practice at the time, these empirical results revealed a more substantial impact of stressors on mental health than was accepted canon at the time.

Finally, although emphasizing the internal workings of the stress process, Pearlin et al. (1981) situated these processes within the organization of society, countering prevailing psychological perspectives that largely ignored the social origins of stressors by treating life events as independent variables.

3.2 The Evolution of the Stress Process

3.2.1 The Structural Context of the Stress Process

Perhaps the most significant turning point in the sociological study of stress was the publication of a paper bearing that title by Pearlin (1989). This manifesto admonished sociologists for ignoring the structural context of the stress process, in particular (1) systems of stratification that cut across society—social and economic class, race/ethnicity, gender, and age; (2) social institutions and their arrangements of statuses and roles; and, (3) interpersonal relationships. These interrelated levels of social structure, Pearlin asserted, mold the experience of individuals and, therefore, are not extraneous to the stress process but are fundamental to it:

> They are the sources of hardship and privilege, threat and security, conflict and harmony. In searching for the origins of stress, we may begin fruitfully by scrutinizing the social arrangements of society and the structuring of experience within these arrangements. This search, I believe, will reveal how ordinary people can be caught up in the disjunctures and discontinuities of society, how they can be motivated to adopt socially valued dreams and yet find their dreams thwarted by socially erected barriers, and how as engaged members of society they come into conflict with others and themselves (Pearlin 1989: 242).

Pearlin went on to declare that sociological stress research should direct its attention to the socially patterned distribution of components of the stress process, focusing on how people's placement in society and participation in social

---

[5] Although the resources of social support and coping were conceptualized as mediators, moderating effects also were hypothesized and tested.

institutions and interpersonal relationships shape: exposure to stressors, access to resources that may influence the impact of stressors, and mental health outcomes.

The social epidemiology of the stress process emerged as one of the discipline's responses to this ground-breaking research agenda (Turner et al. 1995; Turner and Lloyd 1999). This line of research also applied the differential exposure and differential vulnerability hypotheses, which posit, respectively, that the concentration of mental disorder within low status groups can be attributed, at least in part, to disproportionate exposure to stressors, or disproportionate vulnerability to stressors, or both (Kessler 1979a, b). Earlier tests had failed to find much support for the exposure hypothesis, but the life events inventories used in this research were poorly suited to the task for several reasons: (1) the selection of events was arbitrary, such that events occurring to young adults were overrepresented, while those occurring to women, minorities, and the poor were underrepresented (Thoits 1983); (2) stressors that were not eventful had been excluded (Pearlin 1983); and, (3) the exclusion of stressors that might be affected by the person's mental health (to avoid contamination in the measurement of the independent variable by the dependent variable) had the unintended effect of also excluding socially caused stressors, thereby removing the concept of stressors from social structure and processes (Wheaton 1990; Aneshensel 1992). As a result, early tests of the exposure hypothesis were biased in favor of the null hypothesis. The resolution of these issues awaited a reconceptualization of the universe of stressors and an operationalization of it that sampled the full spectrum of stressors to which people are exposed.

3.2.2 The Universe of Stressors

As the limits of life change inventories became apparent (e.g., Thoits 1983), attention increasingly turned to other types of stressors. In counterpoint to the idea that stress resides in change, Pearlin (1983) asserted that it also arises from enduring problems encountered in the enactment of major social roles, such as worker, spouse, and parent. The sources of role strain he identified are: role overload, excessive role demands; role captivity, being an unwilling incumbent of a role, such as caregiver; role restructuring, which occurs when long-standing relationships among members of a role set are renegotiated, for example, adult children providing care for their parents; inter-role conflict, incompatible demands across social roles; and, interpersonal conflict within role sets.

Wheaton (1994) expanded the domain of a chronic stressor beyond role strains to incorporate, for example, barriers in the achievement of life goals; inadequate rewards relative to effort or qualifications; excessive or inadequate environmental demand; frustration of role expectations; and resource deprivation. Other structural sources of chronic stress include inconsistency among dimensions of social status consisting of: status inconsistency—discrepancy between occupation and income, goal-striving stress—discrepancy between aspirations and achievements, and life-style incongruity—consumption patterns and cosmopolitan behaviors inconsistent with social class (Dressler 1988). Overtime, the concept of a chronic stressor has become enlarged further and now includes, for example: enduring interpersonal difficulties; social and economic hardship including poverty, crime, violence, overcrowding, and noise; homelessness, and; chronic physical disability.

As chronic stressors gained traction in stress research, Wheaton (1994) published a description of the "stress universe" that further reoriented thinking about the nature of stressors by expanding its boundaries. The first dimension he distinguishes is the chronicity or *duration* of the stressor, which extends from sudden, one-time unanticipated events to difficulties that are built into everyday life, as illustrated in Fig. 3.2. The second dimension made explicit the idea that stressors occur at multiple *levels* of social organization from (1) the micro-level of the individual and primary social relationships, such as disagreements among co-workers; through (2) the meso- or intermediate-level of organizations and institutions, such as a workplace climate tolerant of sexual harassment; to (3) to the macro-level of society, as exemplified by economic downturns. Most stress research focuses on a single level, usually the micro-level. However, research on macroeconomic factors provides an example of cross-level research, such as studies linking

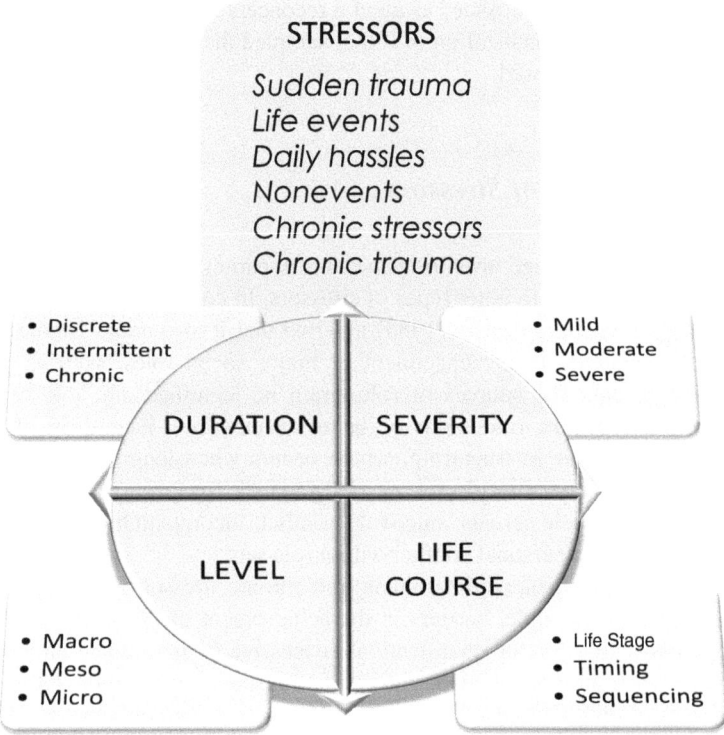

Fig. 3.2 Dimensions of the stress universe. Based on Wheaton (1994) and Wheaton et al. (2013)

recession-induced job insecurity to adverse mental health outcomes even among workers who do not lose their jobs during the recession (see Tausig 2013).

Two additional dimensions also were identified. One is *severity*—how much threat the stressor poses or the extent to which it impedes the attainment of one's goals. The other is a life course dimension, which acknowledges that stressors occurring early in the life course are consequential to mental health later in life, and also that the timing and sequencing of life transitions matters, as when events occur earlier or later than the norm, for instance, early entry into marriage or spousal bereavement in early adulthood (Pearlin and Skaff 1996; Pearlin et al. 2007).

Wheaton (1994) unified an extensive array of distinct types of stressors by locating them within the stress universe and in doing so reset its boundaries. In addition to life change events and chronic stressors, he included several sources of stress that were emergent at the time but not fully integrated into research on the structural contexts of the stress process: traumas, daily hassles, and nonevents. Wheaton et al. (2013) cite the American Psychiatric Association (1987: 250) in describing traumas as stressors of such overwhelming severity that they are "outside the range of usual human experience" and "markedly distressing to almost anyone". Conversely, "daily hassles" are day-to-day irritations and frustrations, such as traffic and waiting in lines (Kanner et al. 1981). Although similar to chronic stressors in their persistent and recurrent nature, daily hassles are distinct in that they are less severe. "Nonevents" are expected or sought-after changes that do not occur, such as being passed over for an anticipated promotion at work (Gersten et al. 1974); they are the mirror opposites of life change events. Current research continues to expand the stress universe, such as several recent examples from non-Western societies including family disruption due to labor out-migration (Lu et al. 2012), food insecurity (Tsai et al. 2012), and large-scale population displacements (Cao et al. 2012).

The dimensions of the stress universe (see Fig. 3.2) can be illustrated with the stressor of perceived discrimination (Harrell 2000; Clark et al. 1999). Discrimination refers to biased behavior toward members of a social group who share an attribute that is devalued and stigmatized in a particular society (Link and Phelan 2001). When conceptualized as a stressor, exposure to discrimination typically is classified into two types (e.g., Williams et al. 1997). The first is major lifetime events, which are discrete incidents of a magnitude sufficient to impact important aspects of a person's life, such as the ability to earn a living, for example, being unfairly denied a promotion. This type of discrimination is usually assessed for any occurrence over the course of one's life. In contrast, everyday experiences of discrimination tend to be repeated or continual and often are ambiguous occurrences, such as receiving poor service at restaurants, and are typically assessed for current experiences. Discrimination occurs at multiple levels, for instance institutional practices like a hiring preference for low wage workers that leads to de facto age discrimination for potentially large numbers of job applicants compared to racial slurs directed at an individual. Most research addresses perceived discrimination at the micro-level, such as a recent study by Grollman (2012) finding that multiple disadvantaged statuses lead to encountering multiple forms of discrimination, which then is associated with worse mental health above the effect of only one form of discrimination. There are exceptions, however, such as Gee's (2002) study of redlining, which is an institutional discriminatory lending practice for mortgages.

As attention focused on the nature of stressors, it became apparent that these sources of stress often are not independent of one another, but instead share a causal connection to one another. Pearlin described these connections as a process of stress proliferation, in which an original or primary stressor leads to a secondary or consequent stressor, which then exerts its own effect on mental health (Pearlin et al. 1997). Proliferation can occur among different types of stressors, for instance: life events can lead to chronic stressors, traumas can result in life events, and so on. For example, Cao et al. (2012) find that the large scale population displacement resulting from China's Three Gorges Dam Project was associated with higher levels of depressive symptoms in part because displacement resulted in a significant decline in living standards.[6] Pearlin and Bierman (2013) argue that stress proliferation directs our attention away from examining one stressor at one particular point in time and toward configurations of multiple stressors occurring at the same time or in a series over time. Failure to fully account for the full spectrum of exposure, they note, may lead to biased estimates of the effect of the primary stressor and may masquerade as differential vulnerability to the primary stressor.

Thus, not only did the boundaries of the stress universe expand, but there was growing awareness that stressors are not necessarily independent occurrences but instead often are woven into the fabric of people's lives. As a result of charting the boundaries and content of the stress universe, it became possible to develop measures that more fully capture the spectrum of stressors to which people may be exposed (e.g., Wheaton 1994; Turner et al. 1995).

Based on these developments, Turner et al. (1995) initiated a line of research on the social epidemiology of the stress process, pursuing the research agenda laid out by Pearlin (1989) as described above. They started by declaring that the differential exposure hypothesis had never been effectively tested because extant research has not used adequate measures of stress exposure (as discussed above). Using a more comprehensive measure, the investigators found that the distribution of stressors varied by social status and that these distributions aligned precisely with that of depressive symptoms and major depressive disorder. Most importantly, differences in exposure accounted for a substantial proportion of the observed status differences in depressive outcomes. Their results also discounted the efficacy of differential vulnerability as an explanation of status differences in depressive outcomes. The investigators concluded that chronic stressors rather than life events are of primary importance to explaining depressive states and their social distributions. It soon became evident that failure to take into account the full

---

[6] Similar indirect effects were found for loss of social integration, which is conceptualized as a secondary stressor, but also could be conceptualized as resources that are depleted by displacement.

array of stressors to which people may be exposed had underestimated the role of stressors in explaining social status differences in depressive symptoms and provided biased estimates of differences in exposure to stressors by race/ethnicity, socioeconomic status, and gender (Avison and Turner 2003).

Related research then considered the extent to which social patterns in personal and social resources exist, and if so, whether these patterns account for parallel patterns in mental disorder, an endeavor that has yielded mixed results. Turner and Marino (1994) found that social support differences by social status parallel the distribution of depressive outcomes (with the exception of gender), but that social support contributes little to the explanation of most status differences in depressive outcomes. Mastery and self-esteem also did little to explain status differences in mental disorder, with the notable exception that the relatively low level of mastery among persons of low SES fully accounts for their tendency to have relatively high levels of depressive outcomes (Turner et al. 1999). Collectively, these results imply that social and personal resources generally do not substantially mediate the association between social status and depressive outcomes; although these resources do have beneficial effects on mental health (see also Turner and Lloyd 1999).

Although existing research has demonstrated that stressors and resources are not distributed randomly but are more concentrated in some social strata than others, the precise nature of these differences and their contribution to explaining social patterns in mental health outcomes continues to be at the forefront of stress research. As a case in point, Boardman et al. (2011) recently examined trajectories of exposure to stressors from adolescence to young adulthood, finding that Blacks have higher rates of exposure than Whites for three of four stress trajectories, including chronic exposure, while Whites have higher rates than Blacks for only one trajectory, being relatively stress free over this time in the life course. However, race differences in exposure accounted for only a modest amount of the higher level of depressive symptoms among Blacks compared to Whites. However, the field has moved away from comprehensive assessments of the influence of multiple stressors in favor of disaggregated studies of single stressors, limiting the extent to which findings are informative about the domain of stressors in general (Wheaton et al. 2013) and the extent to which differential exposure to stressors accounts for status differences in mental health.

Moreover, recent research indicates that high social status is not invariably associated with low exposure to stressors. The stress of higher status hypothesis argues that some desirable characteristics of higher status occupations—such as controlling one's work schedule and working independently—are associated with greater exposure to stressors, such as conflict at the interface between work life and home life (Schieman et al. 2006, 2009; Schieman and Reid 2009) and interpersonal conflict at the workplace (Schieman and Reid 2008, 2009). Similarly, Grzywacz et al. (2004) recently found that better educated persons encounter more frequent daily stressors; however, these stressors were objectively and subjectively less severe, on average, for college graduates than for those with less than a high school degree; and, differential exposure did not account for educational differences in psychological distress.

These exceptions notwithstanding, Thoits (2010) concludes that differential exposure to stress is a central mechanism in generating mental health disparities based on gender, race/ethnicity, marital status, and social class. She also maintains that discrimination is a stressor that adds to the already disproportionately high level of stress exposure among lower status, disadvantaged groups. These same groups generally have lower levels of coping resources too, which means that the groups that could benefit most from resources because of their relatively high exposure to stressors are the same groups that have the least resources.

3.2.3 Outcomes of the Stress Process: A Continuum of Distress Versus Discrete Disorders

Like stressors, the nature of the mental health outcomes of the Stress Process Model also has garnered considerable attention over the years, a particular instance of a larger debate about the most appropriate outcomes for sociological research into mental health, specifically a continuum of psychological distress versus discrete disorder. The latter is based on the medical model, which defines mental disorder as a disease or a disease-like condition that is explained by genetic defects, biochemical imbalances, hormonal dysregulation and neuronal deficits that can be treated through medical means (see Aneshensel et al. 2013). Problematic thoughts, feelings, and actions are seen as signs and symptoms of underlying pathology, and words like mental illness are used literally, not metaphorically. The designation of these states as "signs and symptoms" of a discrete disorder that is either present or absent, such as major depressive disorder, is the quintessence of the medical model.

An alternative perspective, one favored by many sociologists, is that psychopathology is at the extreme negative end of a continuum with similar feelings, thoughts, and behaviors that fall into the realm of normality. Mirowsky and Ross (1989a, b, 2002), staunch critics of the diagnostic approach, argue forcefully that the diagnostic approach impedes scientific understanding by "reifying diagnostic categories", that is, treating observable attributes (such as hallucinations and delusions) as indicators of hypothetical underlying entities (such as Schizophrenia). This practice diverts attention away from the causes of real experiences, they contend, and toward the hidden and possibly nonexistent biological causes of socially constructed psychiatric entities. Mirowsky and Ross (1989a, b, 2002) also have enumerated substantial methodological shortcomings to reducing a measurement of a continuous phenomenon into a dichotomous variable, including: treating everyone who meets diagnostic criteria as if they had the same symptom profile, and ignoring differences in symptomatology among those who do not meet criteria; and, the resulting loss of statistical power that makes it more difficult to detect an association between mental health outcomes and risk factors.

In point and counterpoint, one side of the debate contends that disorder is qualitatively distinct from seemingly similar normal states and that symptom checklists measure "problems in living," which are ephemeral and of limited clinical importance; the other side maintains that diagnostic-type measures trivialize the psychological distress that is most common and consequential in the general population. This debate has been aired in special issues of two journals: *Journal of Health and Social Behavior* (Horwitz 2002a) and *Health: An Interdisciplinary Journal for the Social Study of Health, Illness and Medicine* (Ritter 2007).

In recent years, an arsenal of statistical models—confirmatory factor analysis, latent structural analysis, latent class factor analysis, factor mixture analysis, and growth mixture analysis, and so on—has been applied to symptom data in an attempt of adjudicate this dispute. For instance, taxometric analysis—which uses the distribution and empirical covariation of symptoms to draw inferences about the probable nature of the underlying state as continuous, discrete, or mixed—yields results for symptoms of depression are consistent with both a dimensional model (symptoms of distress, e.g., depressed mood) and a discrete entity (somatic symptoms, e.g. sleeplessness) (Beach and Amir 2003). Although discussion of this issue in sociology has focused on depression and psychological distress, it applies to other conditions as well. For example, van Os and associates (van Os et al. 2009) describe a proneness–persistence–impairment continuum model for psychosis as well as an underlying latent categorical structure, concluding that the population of affected persons may be composed of two types of people. Recent work posits dimensional higher order constructs, such as internalizing and externalizing disorder, for families of discrete disorders with common biological, genetic, environmental, and psychosocial risk factors (Kessler 2013). Although the statistical analysis of quantitative data may yet provide scientific consensus about the nature of disorder, such consensus lies in the future, and many are likely to be persuaded by other criteria, such as the subjective views of the persons who experience these conditions, a position advocated by Mirowsky and Ross (2002)—Descartes versus Locke.

Although the discrete/dimensional debate has been presented at times as an either/or choice, this perspective is inconsistent with the empirical evidence supporting both aspects of mental illness. It seems unnecessarily restrictive to anoint one approach as superior for all sociological research questions, even all studies on the Stress Process Model. A single conceptualization of disorder and mode of assessment simply does not fit all types of inquiries (Aneshensel 2002).

3.2.4 Outcomes of the Stress Process: Single Versus Multiple Outcomes

Research on the stress process historically has emphasized depressive outcomes and continues to do so, although it is now somewhat more common to study multiple outcomes, such as depression and substance abuse. As a result, our knowledge of the mental health consequences of exposure to stressors is thin in comparison to what we know about how stressors function as antecedents of depression. In this regard, Aneshensel et al. (1991) demonstrate that research on a single disorder is inherently inadequate for identifying the overall or total mental health consequences of exposure to stressors. The latter, they argue, requires a dependent variable that captures the full range of disorders for which stress is a plausible etiological factor. When one particular disorder is tacitly treated as a proxy for the universe of all stress-related disorders, people with other stress-related disorders are in essence misclassified because they do not have the disorder under investigation. This misclassification results in biased estimates of the overall effect of stressors on mental health.

An important corollary is that estimates of group differences in the impact of stress for a particular disorder cannot be equated with whether stress exerts a more harmful effect on mental health among some social groups than others, the differential vulnerability hypothesis. Aneshensel et al. (1991) provide an empirical example demonstrating that estimates for two separate disorder-specific models—affective/anxiety and substance-use disorders—are not good approximations of the effect of stressors for a composite category of any psychiatric disorder and provide misleading results with regard to differential vulnerability. Horwitz (2002b) similarly concludes that studying single outcomes misrepresents comparisons of group differences in response to stress when these groups have different psychological responses to stressors, for instance, depression versus substance abuse.

The necessity of examining multiple outcomes is demonstrated by a recent study by Ueno (2010) that applies the stress process model and the minority stress model to explain the relatively high levels of depressive symptoms and drug use among young adults who have had same-sex sexual contact. In this study, stressors and resources contribute to the explanation of the association between sexual minority status and depressive symptoms, but not its association with drug use. Thus, the mental health effects of stressors and resources would have been misrepresented if only depressive symptoms or only drug use had been studied.

Wheaton (2010) enumerates several outcomes that extend beyond mental health to areas of interest to mainstream sociology, including: differential risk for entry into and exits from social roles, such as marriage and divorce; disparity in life outcomes, including those that stem from achievement in the status attainment process, such as attenuated education; differential access to desirable social statuses; and, turning points in the life course. As a concrete example, a recent study by (Boswell et al. 2004) examined the impact of work stress on multiple work outcomes—loyalty, withdrawal from work (e.g., absenteeism), job search, and intent to quit. As another example, Boynton-Jarrett and colleagues (Forthcoming) link "turbulent" life transitions during adolescence—such as frequent residential mobility, school transitions, family structure disruptions, and homelessness—to multiple outcomes in young adulthood including high school completion and cumulative exposure to violence. For these reasons, Wheaton (2010) cites multiple outcomes as a key development in the evolution of the Stress Process Model.

3.3 Future Directions: Mediators and Moderators

Although mediation and moderation figure prominently in research on the stress process, it is our contention that these terms are too often applied in a semi-automatic manner with insufficient attention to the theoretical reasons for why these processes should occur within the context of the types of stressors, resources, and outcomes being studied. Extant research tends to employ a commonsense approach, often post hoc, to explaining why resources act as mediators and/or moderators—as distinct from testing a formal theory about these processes. In particular, we find fault with the application of the concept of mediators as it pertains to the idea that resources *counteract* the mental health effects of stressors because it appears that resources typically do not perform this function. Given this provocative conclusion, some explanation is warranted.

In research on the stress process, mediation typically is inferred when (1) the magnitude of the direct effect of the stressor on the mental health outcome is decreased with the addition of the resource to the model, and (2) the resource has a statistically significant effect on the outcome.[7] This finding, however, does not indicate that the resource counteracts exposure. On the contrary, it shows that the resource is depleted, as when married friends sever ties with couples who divorce, and that the resource is the means through which the stressor exerts its damaging effect on mental health. This dynamic quite clearly runs counter to the idea that the resource counteracts the effects of exposure.

The direct effect of the stressor may instead increase with the addition of a mediator to the model, and it is this pattern that conforms to the idea of resources qua resources. This pattern is the result of a positive sign between the occurrence of the stressor and the resource, indicating mobilization of the resource, for instance, when being fired or laid off from a job prompts former co-workers to help in a job search. Wheaton (1985) identifies this dynamic as an additive form of stress buffering (as distinct from buffering as moderation) because its indirect effect via the resource is opposite to its direct effect such that its total effect is smaller than it would be if the resource had not been activated by the stressor.[8]

Although exceptions exist to the following generalization, studies usually find stress-induced depletion of resources, the opposite of the theoretical function of resources as counteracting stressors. Instead, there are fewer resources when they

---

[7] As noted earlier, the original conceptualization of the Stress Process Model treated self-esteem and mastery as the means through which stressors damage mental health, a conceptualization that evolved over time to the role of resources, perhaps because these concepts, along with social support, do generally counteract the effects of stressors when considered as moderators.

[8] In statistical terms, this is an instance of inconsistent mediation, which means that the indirect effect of the independent variable is opposite in sign to its total effect (MacKinnon 2008). In this case, the indirect pathway from stressors to resources to disorder has a negative sign (+ × − = −) such that an increase in the stressor indirectly produces a decrease in disorder, whereas the total effect of stressors on mental health has a positive sign. Theoretical and analytic neglect of the sign of the relationship between stressors and resources may be the result of the tendency of stress researchers to assess mediation using the difference of coefficients method (instead of the product of coefficients method; MacKinnon 2008), in that it is not necessary to examine the effect of the stressor on the resource. Also, stress researchers often do not test the statistical significance of the mediated effect, an oversight that may lead to the erroneous conclusion that mediation has occurred when it probably has not. Mediation also can be assessed with structural equations models (SEMs), in which case the sign is obvious and tests of statistical significance are parts of the routine output.

are most needed. For instance, Thoits (2013) notes that while self-esteem sometimes increases in response to a stressor, the dominant pattern is decreased self-esteem, leading to the conclusion that the diminishment of self-esteem is one of the pathways through which stressors damage mental health. Our point is not that findings are misinterpreted; this is not the case. Instead, these findings do not seem to have congealed sufficiently to propel the further evolution of the Stress Process Model toward explaining why the depletion of resources occurs more often than mobilization.

At this stage in the evolution of research on the stress process, it is opportune to expand the model to more fully include the theoretical basis for how stressors affect resources and to test these mechanisms. That is, identifying the processes that transmit the effect of the stressor on the resource should become a research objective in its own right. As shown in Fig. 3.3, this elaboration concerns the juncture between stressors and resources, specifically the intermediary factors and processes that mediate mediation.

As an example of the type of theory we have in mind, Thoits (2013) applies symbolic interactionist theory about the derivation and maintenance of self-esteem from perceptions of the reactions of others to the self, including the impact of threats to self-identities on stress appraisal. McLeod's (2013) discussion of social evaluation processes with regard to the impact of social stratification on mental health can be applied to the effects of stressors on resources too. For instance, the application of theory on social comparisons and reference groups to the explanation of why negative appraisals from advantaged groups do not invariably result in low self-esteem among disadvantaged groups is relevant to social psychological processes that might transmit the mental health effects of the types of identity-relevant stressors discussed by Thoits (2013).

Parenthetically, more attention is required regarding the theoretical implications of findings in which hypothesized mediation is not found. In general, these null findings are not addressed sufficiently in favor of interpreting other positive findings of the study. Often these other findings reveal that stressors and resources have separate and opposite effects on the mental health outcome. Wheaton (1985) describes this pattern as an illusory stress-buffering model: Resources offset the stressor, but do not buffer it because the resource operates even in the absence of the stressor. When mediation is hypothesized, these findings disconfirm this aspect of the theory and merit more serious consideration than is often given.

We have parallel observations and recommendations to make about the concept of resources and moderation, although in this instance the idea that resources counteract exposure is merited. In the case of stress-buffering as moderation, the resource plays a protective function, dampening the effect of the stressors relative to having less of the resource. This form of stress-buffering usually is operationalized as a product interaction term between the stressor and the resource. The most firmly established instance of moderation is the stress-buffering function of social support in which exposure to stressors has a stronger adverse effect on mental health among people who derive little support from their social relationships compared to those who feel they are cared for, loved, and esteemed (see Thoits 2011).

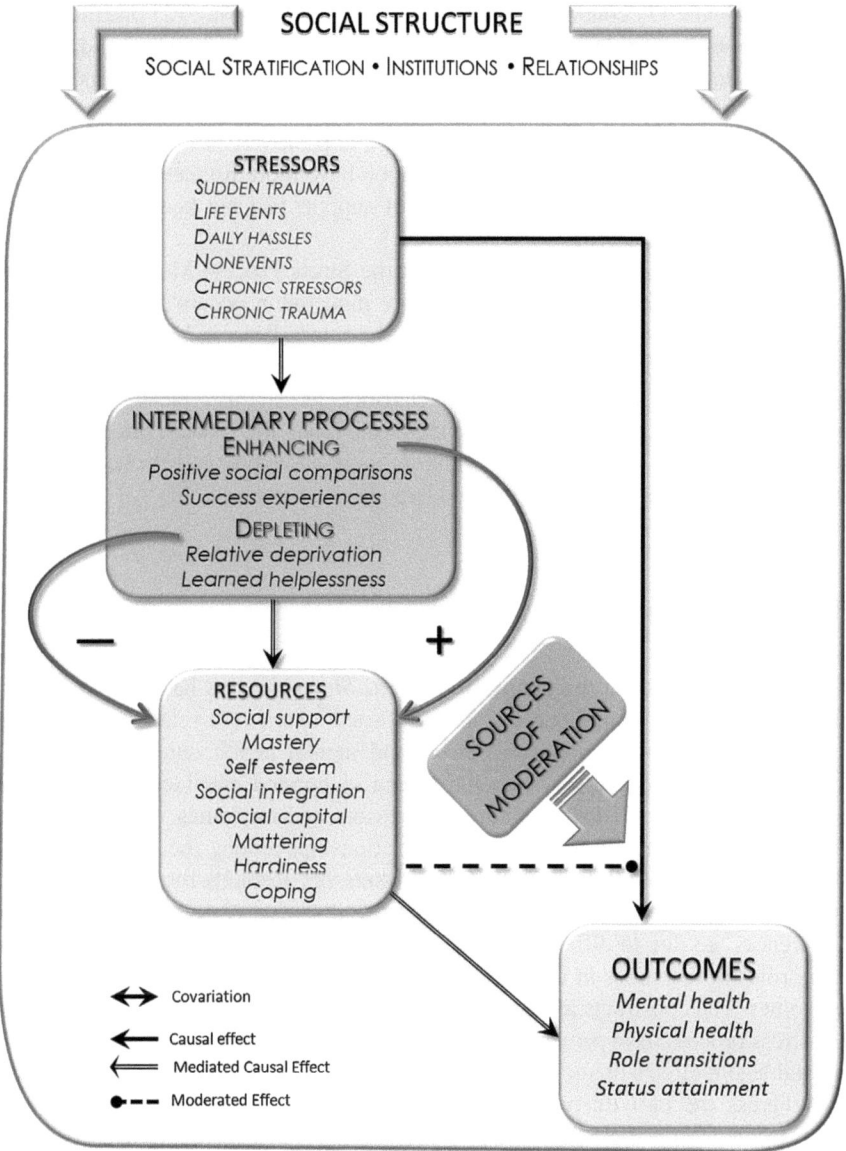

Fig. 3.3 An elaboration of the stress process. Not all paths shown for simplicity

The distinction between mediators and moderators is complicated by the fact that the same resource may serve both functions.

A recent study by Prelow et al. (2006) illustrates these distinctions by testing three models of social support as a mediator and/or moderator of the effect of racial discrimination on depressive symptoms among a sample of African American college students: (1) conditional stress-buffering (moderation), (2) discrimination-induced mobilization of support (mediation as additive buffering); and, (3) the opposite—deterioration of support (mediation opposite to buffering). Findings are consistent with only the support-deterioration model: Discrimination is negatively associated with social support, which, in turn, is positively associated with symptoms so that persons exposed to discrimination have more frequent symptoms than they otherwise would have if their sense of support had not been diminished by exposure to discrimination.

As with mediation, we recommend that the Stress Process Model be expanded to include a theoretical explanation for why moderation occurs and that research test these explanations. This elaboration of the Stress Process Model would entail identifying the factors and processes that account for the effect moderation produced by the resource, as shown in Fig. 3.3. In statistical terms, this typically would mean adding variables to the model that reduce or eliminate the product interaction term that operationalizes moderation. In addition, more attention needs to be paid to the theoretical implications of failing to find hypothesized moderation.

3.4 Conclusions

Earlier we asserted that the publication of *The Stress Process* has been as influential as it has been in large part because it posited a *system* of relationships among stressors, social and personal resources, and mental health outcomes. The constructs that comprise this system have been elaborated considerably over time, especially with regard to the nature of stressors and outcomes. Current applications continue to emphasize several key relationships among these constructs: (1) the extent to which differential exposure to stressors accounts for social status differences in the risk of having a mental health disorder, (2) whether these status differences are due to differential vulnerability, and (3) the mediating and moderating roles of resources in accounting for the effects of exposure on mental health outcomes. The constructs and relationships set forth in the original specification of the stress process have proven to be a solid foundation for subsequent work on the mental health effects of social stress.

Whereas the past thirty years has seen considerable elaboration of the constructs comprising the Stress Process Model, especially stressors, it is our contention that the relationships among these constructs warrants equal attention, specifically the explanation of mediation and the explanation of moderation. This endeavor should flow from the application of mid-range theory about the social origins of self-esteem (see Thoits 2013) and mastery (see Ross and Mirowsky 2013), and the factors that influence the perception of being supported by others (see Turner and Turner 2013). In this regard, we echo Thoits' (2011) recent call for explaining *how* social support exerts its beneficial effects on mental health rather than continuing to demonstrate that it has these effects (although this recommendation pertains to a different juncture in the stress process). Thus, it is our belief that the future of research on the Stress Process Model lies in explicating more fully how this system operates.

The system of relationships set forth in *The Stress Process* (Pearlin et al. 1981) set in motion a program of research carried out by numerous researchers that has elaborated the model's basic constructs and relationships. These developments have illuminated the conceptual overlap with other research areas, especially the life course, social stratification, emotions, and social psychology. In this manner, the Stress Process Model has helped make the sociology of mental health a mainstream area of sociological inquiry.

References

American Psychiatric Association (1987). *Diagnostic and statistical manual of mental disorders*, (3rd ed., text rev). Washington, DC: Author.
Aneshensel, C. S. (1992). Social stress: Theory and research. *Annual Review of Sociology, 18*, 15–38.
Aneshensel, C. S. (2002). Answers and questions in the sociology of mental health. *Journal of Health and Social Behavior, 43*, 236–246.
Aneshensel, C. S., Phelan, J. C., & Bierman, A. (2013). The sociology of mental health: Surveying the field. In C. S. Aneshensel, J. C. Phelan, & A. Bierman (Eds.), *Handbook of the sociology of mental health* (2nd ed., pp. 1–19). Dordrecht: Springer.
Aneshensel, C. S., Rutter, C. M., & Lachenbruch, P. A. (1991). Social structure, stress, and mental health. *American Sociological Review, 56*, 166–179.
Avison, W. R., & Turner, R. J. (1988). Stressful life events and depressive symptoms: Disaggregating the effects of acute stressors and chronic strains. *Journal of Health and Social Behavior, 29*, 253–264.
Avison, W. R., & Turner, R. J. (2003). Status variations in stress exposure: Implications for the interpretation of research on race, socioeconomic status, and gender. *Journal of Health and Social Behavior, 44*, 488–505.
Beach, S. R. H., & Amir, N. (2003). Is depression taxonic, dimensional, or both? *Journal of Abnormal Psychology, 112*, 228–236.
Boardman, J. D., Alexander, K. B., & Stallings, M. C. (2011). Stressful life events and depression among adolescent twin pairs. *Biodemography and Social Biology, 57*, 53–66.
Boswell, W. R., Olson-Buchanan, J. B., & LePine, M. A. (2004). Relations between stress and work outcomes: The role of felt challenge, job control, and psychological strain. *Journal of Vocational Behavior, 64*, 165–181.
Boynton-Jarrett, R., Hair, E., & Zuckerman, B. (Forthcoming). Turbulent times: Effect of turbulence and violence exposure in adolescence on high school completion, health risk behavior, and mental health in young adulthood. *Social Science and Medicine*.
Cao, Y., Hwang, S.-S., & Xi, J. (2012). Project-induced displacement, secondary stressors, and health. *Social Science and Medicine, 74*, 1130–1138.
Clark, R., Anderson, N. B., Clark, V. R., & Williams, D. R. (1999). Racism as a stressor for African Americans: A biopsychosocial model. *American Psychologist, 54*, 805–816.
Dohrenwend, B. S., Krasnoff, L., Askenasy, A. R., & Dohrenwend, B. P. (1978). Exemplification of a method for scaling life events: The PERI life events scale. *Journal of Health and Social Behavior, 19*, 205–229.
Dressler, W. W. (1988). Social consistency and psychological distress. *Journal of Health and Social Behavior, 29*, 79–91.
Gee, G. C. (2002). A multilevel analysis of the relationship between institutional and individual racial discrimination and health status. *American Journal of Public Health, 92*, 615–623.

Gersten, J. C., Langner, T. S., Eisenberg, J. G., & Orzeck, L. (1974). Child behavior and life events: Undesirable change or change per se? In B. S. Dohrenwend & B. P. Dohrenwend (Eds.), *Stressful life events: Their nature and effects* (pp. 159–170). New York: Wiley.

Glavin, P., Schieman, S., & Reid, S. (2011). Boundary-spanning work demands and their consequences for guilt and psychological distress. *Journal of Health and Social Behavior, 52*, 43–57.

Glover, D. A. (2006). Allostatic load in women with and without PTSD symptoms. *Annuals of the New York Academy of Sciences, 1071*, 442–447.

Grollman, E. A. (2012). Multiple forms of perceived discrimination and health among adolescents and young adults. *Journal of Health and Social Behavior, 53*, 199–214.

Grzywacz, J. G., Almeida, D. M., Neupert, S. D., & Ettner, S. L. (2004). Socioeconomic status and health: A micro-level analysis of exposure and vulnerability to daily stressors. *Journal of Health and Social Behavior, 45*, 1–10.

Harrell, S. P. (2000). A multidimensional conceptualization of racism-related stress: Implications for the well-being of people of color. *American Journal of Orthopsychiatry, 70*, 42–57.

Horwitz, A. V. (Ed.). (2002a). Selecting outcomes for the sociology of mental health: Issues of measurement and dimensionality [Special issue]. *Journal of Health and Social Behavior, 43*.

Horwitz, A. V. (2002b). Outcomes in the sociology of mental health and illness: Where have we been and where are we going. *Journal of Health and Social Behavior, 43*, 143–151.

Kanner, A. D., Coyne, J. C., Schaefer, C., & Lazarus, R. S. (1981). Comparison of two modes of stress measurement: Daily hassles and uplifts versus major life events. *Journal of Behavioral Medicine, 4*, 1–39.

Karlamanga, A. S., Singer, B. H., McEwen, B. S., Rowe, J. W., & Seeman, T. E. (2002). Allostatic load as a predictor of functional decline MacArthur studies of successful aging. *Journal of Clinical Epidemiology, 55*, 696–710.

Kessler, R. C. (1979a). A strategy for studying differential vulnerability to the psychological consequences of stress. *Journal of Health and Social Behavior, 20*, 100–108.

Kessler, R. C. (1979b). Stress, social status, and psychological distress. *Journal of Health and Social Behavior, 20*, 259–272.

Kessler, R. C. (2013). Overview of descriptive epidemiology of mental disorders. In C. S. Aneshensel, J. C. Phelan, & A. Bierman (Eds.), *Handbook of the sociology of mental health* (2nd ed., pp. 169–182). Dordrecht: Springer.

Lazarus, R. S. (1966). *Psychological stress and the coping process*. New York: McGraw-Hill.

Link, B. G., & Phelan, J. C. (2001). Social conditions as fundamental causes of disease. *Journal of Health and Social Behavior, 35*, 80–94.

Lu, Y., Peifeng, H., & Treiman, D. J. (2012). Migration and depressive symptoms in migrant-sending areas: Findings from the survey of internal migration and health in China. *International Journal of Public Health, 57*, 691–698.

MacKinnon, D. P. (2008). *Introduction of statistical mediation analysis*. New York: Taylor & Francis Group.

McEwen, B. S., & Stellar, E. (1993). Stress and the individual. *Archives of Internal Medicine, 153*, 2093–2101.

McLeod, J. (2013). Social stratification and inequality. In C. S. Aneshensel, J. C. Phelan, & A. Bierman (Eds.), *Handbook of the sociology of mental health* (2nd ed., pp. 229–253). Dordrecht: Springer.

Menaghan, E. G. (1983). Individual coping effects: Moderators of the relationship between life stress and mental health outcomes. In H. B. Kaplan (Ed.), *Psychosocial stress: Trends in theory and research* (pp. 157–191). New York: Academic Press Inc.

Mirowsky, J., & Ross, C. E. (1989a). Psychiatric diagnosis as reified measurement. *Journal of Health and Social Behavior, 30*, 11–25.

Mirowsky, J., & Ross, C. E. (1989b). Rejoinder—assessing the type and severity of psychological problems: An alternative to diagnosis. *Journal of Health and Social Behavior, 30*, 38–40.

Mirowsky, J., & Ross, C. E. (2002). Measurement for a human science. *Journal of Health and Social Behavior, 43*, 152–170.

Pearlin, L. I. (1983). Role strains and personal stress. In H. B. Kaplan (Ed.), *Psychosocial stress: Trends in theory and research* (pp. 3–32). New York: Academic Press Inc.

Pearlin, L. I. (1989). The sociological study of stress. *Journal of Health and Social Behavior, 30*, 241–256.

Pearlin, L. I., & Aneshensel, C. S. (1986). Coping and social supports: Their functions and applications. In L. H. Aiken & D. Mechanic (Eds.), *Applications of social science to clinical medicine and health policy* (pp. 417–437). New Brunswick: Rutgers University Press.

Pearlin, L. I., Aneshensel, C. S., & LeBlanc, A. J. (1997). The Forms and mechanisms of stress proliferation: The case of aids caregivers. *Journal of Health and Social Behavior, 38*, 223–236.

Pearlin, L. I., & Bierman, A. (2013). Current issues and future directions in research into the stress process. In C. S. Aneshensel, J. C. Phelan, & A. Bierman (Eds.), *Handbook of the sociology of mental health* (2nd ed., pp. 325–340). Dordrecht: Springer.

Pearlin, L. I., Menaghan, E. G., Lieberman, M. A., & Mullan, J. T. (1981). The stress process. *Journal of Health and Social Behavior, 22*, 337–356.

Pearlin, L. I., Nguyen, K. B., Schieman, S., & Milkie, M. A. (2007). The life-course origins of mastery among older people. *Journal of Health and Social Behavior, 48*, 164–179.

Pearlin, L. I., & Schooler, C. (1978). The structure of coping. *Journal of Health and Social Behavior, 19*, 2–21.

Pearlin, L. I., & Skaff, M. M. (1996). Stress and the life course: A paradigmatic alliance. *The Gerontologist, 36*, 239–247.

Prelow, H. M., Mosher, C. E., & Bowman, M. A. (2006). Perceived racial discrimination, social support, and psychological adjustment among African American students. *Journal of Black Psychology, 32*, 442–454.

Rabkin, J. G., & Struening, E. L. (1976). Life events, stress, and illness. *Science, 194*, 1013–1020.

Ritter, C. (Ed.) (2007). An introduction to a dialogue about psychological distress and mental disorder. [Special issue]. *Health: An Interdisciplinary Journal for the Social Study of Health, Illness and Medicine, 11*.

Ross, C. E., & Mirowsky, J. (1979). A comparison of life-event weighting schemes: Change, undesirability, and effect-proportional indices. *Journal of Health and Social Behavior, 20*, 166–177.

Ross, C. E., & Mirowsky, J. (2013). The sense of personal control: Social structural causes and emotional consequences. In C. S. Aneshensel, J. C. Phelan, & A. Bierman (Eds.), *Handbook of the sociology of mental health* (2nd ed., pp. 379–402). Dordrecht: Springer.

Schieman, S., Milkie, M. A., & Glavin, P. (2009). When work interferes with life: Work-nonwork interference and the influence of work-related demands and resources. *American Sociological Review, 74*, 966–988.

Schieman, S., & Reid, S. (2008). Job authority and interpersonal conflict in the workplace. *Work and Occupations, 35*, 296–326.

Schieman, S., & Reid, S. (2009). Job authority and health: Unraveling the competing suppression and explanatory influences. *Social Science and Medicine, 69*, 1616–1624.

Schieman, S., Whitestone, Y. K., & Van Gundy, K. (2006). The nature of work and the stress of higher status. *Journal of Health and Social Behavior, 47*, 242–257.

Seeman, T. E., Crimmins, E., Huang, M.-H., Singer, B., Bucur, A., Gruenewald, T., et al. (2004). Cumulative biological risk and socio-economic differences in mortality: MacArthur studies of successful aging. *Social Science and Medicine, 58*, 1985–1997.

Selye, H. (1936). A syndrome produced by diverse nocuous agents. *Nature, 138*, 32.

Smith, W. K. (1987). The stress analogy. *Schizophrenia Bulletin, 13*, 215–220.

Tausig, Mark. (2013). The sociology of work and well-being. In C. S. Aneshensel, J. C. Phelen, & A. Bierman (Eds.), *Handbook of the Sociology of Mental Health* (2nd ed., pp. 433–455). Dordrecht: Springer.

Thoits, P. A. (1983). Dimensions of life events that influence psychological distress: An evaluation and synthesis of the literature. In H. B. Kaplan (Ed.), *Psychosocial stress: Trends in theory and research* (pp. 33–103). New York: Academic Press Inc.

Thoits, P. A. (2010). Stress and health: Major findings and policy implications. *Journal of Health and Social Behavior, 51*, S41–S53.
Thoits, P. A. (2011). Mechanisms linking social ties and support to physical and mental health. *Journal of Health and Social Behavior, 52*, 145–161.
Thoits, P. A. (2013). Self, identity, stress, and mental health. In C. S. Aneshensel, J. C. Phelan, & A. Bierman (Eds.), *Handbook of the sociology of mental health* (2nd ed., pp. 357–377). Dordrecht: Springer.
Tsai, A. C., Bangsberg, D. R., Frongillo, E. A., Hunt, P. W., Muzoora, C., Martin, J. N., et al. (2012). Food insecurity, depression and the modifying role of social support among people living with HIV/AIDS in rural Uganda. *Social Science and Medicine, 74*, 2012–2019.
Turner, R. J., & Lloyd, D. A. (1999). The stress process and the social distribution of depression. *Journal of Health and Social Behavior, 40*, 374–404.
Turner, R. J., Lloyd, D. A., & Roszell, P. (1999). Personal resources and the social distribution of depression. *American Journal of Community Psychology, 27*, 643–672.
Turner, R. J., & Marino, F. (1994). Social support and structure: A descriptive epidemiology. *Journal of Health and Social Behavior, 35*, 193–212.
Turner, J. B., & Turner, R. J. (2013). Social relations, social integration, and social support. In C. S. Aneshensel, J. C. Phelan, & A. Bierman (Eds.), *Handbook of the sociology of mental health* (2nd ed., pp. 341–356). Dordrecht: Springer.
Turner, R. J., Wheaton, B., & Lloyd, D. A. (1995). The epidemiology of social stress. *American Sociological Review, 60*, 104–125.
Ueno, K. (2010). Mental health differences between young adults with and without same-sex contact: A simultaneous examination of underlying mechanisms. *Journal of Health and Social Behavior, 51*, 391–407.
van Os, J., Linscott, R. J., Myin-Germeys, I., Delespaul, P., & Krabbendam, L. (2009). A systematic review and meta-analysis of the psychosis continuum: Evidence for a psychosis proneness-persistence-impairment model of psychotic disorder. *Psychological Medicine, 39*, 179–195.
Wheaton, B. (1985). Models for the stress-buffering functions of coping resources. *Journal of Health and Social Behavior, 26*, 352–364.
Wheaton, B. (1990). Life transitions, role histories, and mental health. *American Sociological Review, 55*, 209–224.
Wheaton, B. (1994). Sampling the stress universe. In W. R. Avison & I. H. Gotlib (Eds.), *Stress and mental health: Contemporary issues and prospects for the future* (pp. 77–114). New York: Plenum Press.
Wheaton, B. (2010). The stress process as a successful paradigm. In W. R. Avison, C. S. Aneshensel, S. Schieman, & B. Wheaton (Eds.), *Advances in the conceptualization of the stress process: Essays in honor of Leonard I. Pearlin* (pp. 231–252). New York: Springer.
Wheaton, B., Young, M., Montazer, S., & Stuart-Lahman, K. (2013). Social stress in the Twenty-First Century. In C. S. Aneshensel, J. C. Phelan, & A. Bierman (Eds.), *Handbook of the sociology of mental health* (2nd ed., pp. 299–323). Dordrecht: Springer.
Williams, D. R., Yan, Y., Jackson, J. S., & Anderson, N. B. (1997). Racial differences in physical and mental health: Socio-economic status, stress and discrimination. *Journal of Health Psychology, 2*, 335–351.

Chapter 4
Mental Illness Stigma and the Sociology of Mental Health

Bruce G. Link and Jo C. Phelan

Scanning the development of research pertaining to labeling and stigma as it pertains to mental illnesses over the past 30 years reveals a deep connection between these fields of inquiry and the development of the American Sociological Association's Section on the Sociology of Mental Health. As research in this domain progressed, the need for a specific home for that research within the ASA became apparent, and as the section grew and supported sessions specifically on labeling and stigma this domain of research was further enhanced. At this juncture sociological understandings of labeling and stigma stand as one of the major successes of the section on the Sociology of Mental Illness. The work has linked the section to the broader discipline through papers published in The American Sociological Review and the American Journal of Sociology and has also brought critical sociological perspectives to relevant disciplines of anthropology, psychology, psychiatry and public health. We seek to capture some of these developments and the impact they have had on understanding the social context of mental illness. Our focus, like the focus of the volume, has been on contributions emanating from the sociology of mental health and consequently we pay less attention to the large advances that have been made in other disciplines, especially anthropology (e.g. Parker and Aggleton 2003; Yang et al. 2007) and social psychology (see Major and O'Brien 2005). Specifically, we point to conceptual advances, studies of public conceptions of mental illnesses, and research that pertains to how people are affected by stigma. We begin with some selected observations about the background of research in this area that help set the stage for understanding some of the advances that have been made in recent years.

B.G. Link (✉) · J.C. Phelan
Columbia University, New York, NY, USA
e-mail: BGL1@Columbia.edu

J.C. Phelan
e-mail: JCP13@Columbia.edu

4.1 Background

Before Goffman's book, *Stigma: Notes on the Management of Spoiled Identity*, the term stigma was used in the social sciences to mean something quite close to its current meaning but was used only infrequently. A Google Scholar search for the period 1900–1960 returns numerous scientific articles using the term "stigma" but almost all of these refer to botany (the receptive apex of the pistil of a flower) or other biological phenomena (a small mark, spot, or pore) rather than to social science meanings of the term. A Google Scholar search in the current era reveals something entirely different with the social science meaning of the term ascendant and being applied to a vast array of stigmatizing circumstances. Another indicator of the large increase in interest is the number of published articles with the word "stigma" in the title or abstract. In 1980 the number stood at 19 for Medline and 14 for Psych Info, but rose dramatically by the end of the century to 114 for Medline and 161 for Psych Info in 1999 (Link and Phelan 2001). Incredibly, by 2010 the numbers were more than five times as high as in 1999: 758 for Medline and 851 for Psych Info. Of course not all of these referred to mental illness stigma but many did and there is no doubt that this trend concerning stigma in general has also applied to mental illness stigma in particular.

4.1.1 Origins: Goffman and the Labeling Debate

In the mid 1950s, Erving Goffman was a research fellow at the Laboratory for Social and Environmental Studies at the National Institute of Mental Health. The unit was headed at the time by sociologist John Clausen, and it was during this period that Goffman did his ethnographic work *Asylums* at Saint Elizabeth's Hospital (Goffman 1961). Stigma was on the minds of the small but enormously generative group at the Laboratory for Social and Environmental Studies, especially in the context of qualitative studies they were undertaking concerning wives of men who were hospitalized for mental illness. Whereas the term stigma was not in wide use in the social sciences at the time, one exception was a paper from this group authored by Schwartz (1956) entitled "The Stigma of Mental Illness." She indicated that stigma had "two connotations: first, that in the minds of others the person is set apart—that is, different from the so-called normal person; second that he is set apart by a 'mark' which is felt to be 'disgraceful,' or even 'immoral,' by which he can be judged to be 'inferior'" (Schwartz 1956, p. 7). Exposed to these ideas and drawing on his ethnography in Saint Elizabeth's hospital, Goffman (1961) produced his highly influential introduction to the stigma concept. Goffman's (1963) description was comprehensive, and it is difficult to find any current consideration of the concept that is not foreshadowed in his 1963 treatise. It is in this work that perhaps the most influential definition of the concept was provided: "an attribute that is deeply discrediting" and that reduces the bearer "from a whole and usual person to a tainted, discounted one" (Goffman 1963, p. 3).

Subsequent to its introduction stigma played a central role in the so-called labeling debate that emerged during the 1960s. Scheff (1966) constructed a formal labeling theory of mental illness that located the origin of stable mental illness in societal reactions including stigmatizing reactions. The essence of his theory is captured in the following quote:

> In a crisis, when the deviance of an individual becomes a public issue, the traditional stereotype of insanity becomes the guiding imagery for action, both for those reacting to the deviant and, at times, for the deviant himself. When societal agents and persons around the deviant react to him uniformly in terms of the stereotypes of insanity, his amorphous and unstructured rule-breaking tends to crystallize in conformity to these expectations, thus becoming similar to behavior of other deviants classified as mentally ill and stable over time. The process of becoming uniform and stable is completed when the traditional imagery becomes a part of the deviant's orientation for guiding his own behavior (Scheff 1966, p. 82).

The theory is called "labeling" theory because of the centrality it gave to social definition of deviant behaviors. The debate concerning the role of labeling in mental illness involved both informal labeling processes (e.g. spouses labeling of their partners) and official labeling through treatment contact (e.g. psychiatric hospitalization). In Scheff's theory, the act of labeling was strongly influenced by the social characteristics of the labelers, the person being labeled, and by the social situation in which their interactions occurred. He asserted that labeling was driven as much by these social factors as it was by anything that might be called the symptoms of mental illness. Moreover, according to Scheff, once a person is labeled, powerful social forces come into play to encourage a stable pattern of "mental illness." Stigma was a central process in this theory as it "punished" people who sought to shed the identity of mental illness and return to normal social roles, interactions and identities.

Critics of the theory, especially Walter Gove, took sharp issue with Scheff's characterization of the labeling process. Gove argued that labels are applied far less capriciously and with many fewer untoward consequences than claimed by labeling theorists (Gove 1975). For some period between the late 1970s and early 1980s, professional opinion swayed in favor of the critics of labeling theory. Certainly the dominant view during that time was that stigma associated with mental illness was relatively inconsequential. Gove for example, concluded that "… stigma appears to be transitory and does not appear to pose a severe problem" (Gove 1982, p. 290) and Crocetti and Spiro (1974) concluded that "former patients enjoy nearly total acceptance in all but the most intimate relationships." Moreover, when a group of expert stigma researchers was summoned to the National Institute of Mental Health in 1980 to review evidence about the issue, the term "stigma" was intentionally omitted from the title of the proceedings. Apparently, the argument that behaviors rather than labels are the prime determinants of social rejection was so forcefully articulated that the editors of the proceedings decided that stigma was not an appropriate designation when "one is referring to negative attitudes induced by manifestations of psychiatric illness" (Rabkin 1984, p. 327). It was within this context that so-called "modified labeling theory" (described in some detail below) emerged in response to the then dominant anti-labeling, stigma-dismissing stance that characterized the field at the time. In the ensuing years major advances in concepts, measures and empirical assessments of mental illness stigma unfolded, many within the context of the Section on the Sociology of Mental Health.

4.2 Conceptualizing Stigma

4.2.1 What Is Stigma?

In the literature on stigma, the term has been used to describe what seem to be quite different concepts. It has been used to refer to the "mark" or "label" that is used as a social designation, to the linking of the label to negative stereotypes, or to the propensity to exclude or otherwise discriminate against the designated person. Even Goffman's (1963) famous essay includes several somewhat different, albeit very instructive, definitions. As a consequence of this variability, there has been confusion as to what the term means. Additionally, an intense dissatisfaction with the concept emerged in some circles for at least two reasons. First, it was argued that the stigma concept identifies an "attribute" or a "mark" as residing in the person—something the person possesses. The objection to this conceptualization was that it took for granted the process of affixing labels and did not interrogate the social processes that led to such labeling (Fine and Asche 1988). In particular, far too little attention had been focused on the selection of a single characteristic for social salience from a vast range of possible characteristics that might have been identified instead. Second, it was argued that too much emphasis had been placed on cognitive processes of category formation and stereotyping and too little on the broad and very prominent fact of discrimination and the influence that such discrimination has on the distribution of life chances (Oliver 1992).

In light of this confusion and controversy, Link and Phelan (2001) put forward a definition of stigma that recognized the overlap in meaning between concepts like stigma, labeling, stereotyping and discrimination. This conceptualization defined stigma in the relationship *between* interrelated components. The idea to do this followed an insight from Goffman who at one point indicated that the essence of stigma lay in the *relationship* between an attribute and a stereotype. As described below, this conceptualization defines stigma in the co-occurrence of interrelated components of labeling, stereotyping, separating, emotional reactions, status loss and discrimination. The approach also responds to the criticism that the stigma concept locates the "mark" or "attribute" in the person by making it clear that such "marks" (or "labels" as designated by Link and Phelan) are selected for social salience from among many possible human traits that might have been selected. This approach also responds to prior criticisms by making the social selection of designations a prominent feature, by incorporating discrimination into the concept, and by focusing on the importance of social, economic and political power in the production of stigma. Link and Phelan describe their conceptualization as follows:

> In our conceptualization, stigma exists when the following interrelated components converge. In the first component, people distinguish and label human differences. In the

second, dominant cultural beliefs link labeled persons to undesirable characteristics—to negative stereotypes. In the third, labeled persons are placed in distinct categories so as to accomplish some degree of separation of "us" from "them." In the fourth, labeled persons experience status loss and discrimination that lead to unequal outcomes. Stigmatization is entirely contingent on access to social, economic and political power that allows the identification of differentness, the construction of stereotypes, the separation of labeled persons into distinct categories and the full execution of disapproval, rejection, exclusion and discrimination. Thus we apply the term stigma when elements of labeling, stereotyping, separation, status loss and discrimination co-occur in a power situation that allows them to unfold (Link and Phelan 2001, p. 367).

A detailed exposition of each of these components is available elsewhere (Link and Phelan 2001, 2012). Here we provide a brief description of each component, connecting each component to the stigma associated with mental illness (although they are intended to be applicable to other stigmatized circumstances as well).

Distinguishing and labeling differences. The vast majority of human differences, e.g., eye color, favorite ice cream or ear lobe width, are not considered to be socially relevant bases for constructing sharp group boundaries. However, some differences, such as skin color and sexual preferences, are currently awarded a high degree of social salience. Both the selection of salient characteristics and the creation of labels for them are social achievements that must be present for stigma to exist. In the area of mental illnesses The *Diagnostic and Statistical Manual of Mental Disorders* (DSM) of the American Psychiatric Association represents an attempt by professionals to decide which human differences should be selected for designation as mental illnesses and which should not. This social selection of human differences and social production of designations is particularly apparent when the criteria are contested, as they were when homosexuality was removed from the DSM, and as they are now with respect to whether or not normal human emotional states such as sadness are being pathologized (Horwitz and Wakefield 2007).

Associating differences with negative attributes. In this component, the labeled difference is linked to negative stereotypes. For example, one common stereotype is that a person who has been hospitalized for mental illness is likely to be unpredictable. Other powerful stereotypes associated with mental illnesses involve inferences about competence, dangerousness, cleanliness and trustworthiness. In the Link and Phelan conceptualization, stereotypes like these must be present and operative for stigma to exist—there must be some linking of a label to a stereotype.

Separating *"us" from "them"*. Central to early and nearly all definitions of stigma (e.g. Jones et al. 1984; Schwartz 1956) a third aspect of the stigma process occurs when labels connote a separation of "us" from "them." Examples can be found with respect to certain ethnic or national groups (Morone 1997), people with mental illness, or people with a different sexual orientation who may be considered fundamentally different kinds of people from "us." In the area of mental illness such a separation is sometimes embedded in the language we use to describe people. For example a person has heart disease, cancer or an infection but a person who develops schizophrenia *"is"* a *"schizophrenic"*—a different sort of person than the rest of "us."

Emotional Responses. The Link and Phelan conceptualization of stigma subsequently was expanded to include emotional responses. Link et al. (2004) noted that from the vantage point of a stigmatizer, emotions of anger, irritation, anxiety, pity and fear are likely. From the vantage point of the person who is stigmatized, emotions of embarrassment, shame, fear, alienation or anger are possible.

Status loss and discrimination. When people are labeled, set apart and linked to undesirable characteristics, a rationale is constructed for devaluing, rejecting and excluding them. When devaluation, discrimination and exclusion are widespread, a persistent pattern of unequal social relationships arises that creates social structures of disadvantage. Once in place these structural arrangements (segregation, exclusion, downward occupational placement) feedback to reinvigorate the labels, stereotypes, setting apart and emotional reactions that disadvantage stigmatized groups.

The dependence of stigma on power. A unique feature of Link and Phelan's (2001) definition is the idea that stigma is entirely dependent on social, cultural, economic and political power. Lower-power groups (e.g., mental health consumers) may label, stereotype and separate themselves from higher-power groups (e.g., psychiatrists) by perhaps labeling the psychiatrists "pill pushers," stereotyping them as "cold" "haughty," and "clueless" and seeing them as a separate group that is distinct from "us." But in this case, stigma as we define it does not exist, because the potentially stigmatizing group (the mental health consumers) do not have the social, cultural, economic and political power to imbue their cognitions (labels and stereotypes) with serious discriminatory consequences. The psychiatrists are not severely damaged materially by the consumers' stereotypes about them. Stigma is dependent on power.

4.2.1.1 Why Do People Stigmatize?

Whereas the Link and Phelan (2001) conceptualization provided concepts that help us to understand what stigma is, the scheme does not tell us why people stigmatize nor why mental illnesses might be stigmatized. Filling this gap Phelan et al. (2008) provide a conceptual scheme that addresses the issue of why people stigmatize. The essence of the answer they provide is that stigmatizing helps people attain ends they desire. They propose three generic ends that people can attain by stigmatizing others: (1) exploitation/domination or *keeping people down*, (2) enforcement of social norms or *keeping people in*, and (3) avoidance of disease or *keeping people away*. We briefly review these reasons for stigmatization and then use them to consider why mental illnesses might be stigmatized.

Exploitation and domination. Wealth, power, and high social status can be attained when one group dominates or exploits another. Ideologies involving stigmatization develop to legitimate and perpetuate these inequalities with the group designated as the one to be kept down being deemed to be inferior in terms of intelligence, character, competence and the basic human qualities of worthiness, and value (Phelan et al. 2008). Classic examples are the racial stigmatization of

African Americans beginning in the era of slavery, the Europeans' colonization of countries around the globe, and U.S. whites' expropriation of the lands of American Indians (Feagin 2009).

Enforcement of social norms. People construct a labyrinth of written and unwritten rules governing everything from how nation states should wage war to how a New Yorker should make it into a subway car. Some degree of investment in norms like these develops; people come to count on them and to be outraged or annoyed when they are violated. Failure to comply with these norms is often cast in terms of the flawed morality or character of the transgressor (Goffman 1963; Morone 1997), and stigma processes are deployed as a corrective mechanism. One way that stigma is useful, then, is that it imparts a stiff cost—a strong social disapproval—that can make subsequent transgressions less likely. In this use of stigma, people are *kept in* by influencing the behavior of the norm violator. A related use is that the people around the norm violator are *kept in* by learning the boundaries of acceptable behavior and by observing the stern example of what happens to someone who goes beyond those bounds (Erikson 1966).

Avoidance of disease. Many illnesses and disabilities (e.g. HIV, facial disfigurement, limb loss) are probably not stigmatized in order to exploit or dominate or in order to directly control behavior and enforce norms. Kurzban and Leary (2001) provide another explanation for stigma in these circumstances by arguing that there are evolutionary pressures to avoid members of one's species who may spread disease. They focus on parasites noting that infection can lead to "deviations from the organism's normal (healthy) phenotype" (Kurzban and Leary 2001, p. 197) such as asymmetry, marks, lesions and discoloration; coughing, sneezing and excretion of fluids; and behavioral anomalies due to damage to muscle-control systems. They argue that the advantage of avoiding disease might have led to a more general aversion to deviations from any local standard for the way humans are supposed to look or carry themselves (Kurzban and Leary 2001). Thus a broad band of deviations might lead to a visceral response of disgust and a strong desire to keep the person with the deviation away.

Why do people stigmatize mental illnesses? In keeping with the strong emphasis in sociological thinking about "residual rule breaking" (Scheff 1966) and the extension of that thinking through the sociology of emotions to "feeling rules" (Thoits 1985), we believe that the major reason for the stigmatization of people with mental illnesses is an attempt to *keep people in*. Initial reactions to symptoms are generally common-sense attempts to rein in the rule-breaking behavior by strongly disapproving of odd beliefs expressed by people with psychosis, admonishing a person with depression to "snap out of it," or passing favorite foods into the sight lines of a person with anorexia. At the same time, the bizarre behavior of psychosis; the weight loss, enervation, and anhedonia of depression; or the extreme underweight associated with anorexia could stimulate a desire for "disease avoidance." Although there is little reason to suppose that mental illnesses are stigmatized so that those who suffer from them can be exploited or dominated for pecuniary gain when efforts to keep people in fail, *keeping people away* can be substituted as a strategy to avoid non-normative behavior. And to the extent that keeping people away is more easily achieved when people are relatively powerless, we might expect that *keeping people down* would also be prominent in the case of serious mental illnesses. Thus we expect a strong initial motivation to stigmatize mental illnesses resides in efforts to keep people in, but when symptomatic behaviors endure and efforts to keep people in fail, motivations to keep people down and away are also evident.

4.2.2 Stigma Power: People's Use of Stigma to Achieve Desired Ends

A novel feature of the Link and Phelan definition of stigma (described above) is the incorporation of "power" in that definition. Successful stigmatization requires power; it requires the ability to construct stereotypes that are broadly endorsed and deeply held; and it requires control over jobs, housing, and education to enact discriminatory behavior that has teeth. Thus, it "takes power" to stigmatize.

However, in light of Phelan et al.'s (2008) consideration of the reasons people stigmatize, we now realize that people achieve outcomes they desire when they stigmatize others. Whether the motive is to *keep people down*, *keep people in* or *keep people away*, stigma is a useful instrument to accomplish ends that are congenial to the stigmatizer's interests. Conceived in this way, stigma is a *source of power* that helps the stigmatizer control the stigmatized person and thereby keep them down, in or away. Thus, we now take the idea that it "takes power" to stigmatize and add the notion that stigmatization confers power—"stigma power."

The concept of stigma power can be thought of as one form of what Bourdieu called "symbolic power." For Bourdieu (1987), symbolic power is the capacity to impose on others a legitimatized vision of the social world and of the cleavages within that world. Bourdieu developed and used the concept mainly to understand class and class reproduction, adding a cultural element to the understanding of those phenomena. But three aspects of Bourdieu's concept are extremely useful with regard to understanding stigma and the power it confers. First, cultural distinctions of value and worth are the critically important mechanisms through which power is exercised. Stigma is in many respects a statement about value and worth made by a stigmatizer about those he or she might stigmatize and, thus, one form of symbolic power in Bourdieu's terms. Second, those who are disadvantaged by the exercise of power are often persuaded, sometimes without realizing it, to accept as valid the cultural evaluations that harm them. Finally, the exercise of symbolic power is often buried in taken-for-granted aspects of culture and thereby hidden, or "misrecognized" as Bourdieu (1990) put it, by both the people causing the harm and by those being harmed.

To explore the utility of the stigma power concept with respect to mental illnesses, Link and Phelan (2014) examined ways in which the goals of stigmatizers are achieved but hidden in the stigma coping efforts of people with mental illnesses. Capitalizing on new measures from a small study of stigma and psychosis,

Link and Phelan found that people with psychosis are aware of the cultural assessment of their lower social standing, show a high degree of concern about staying within normative boundaries, an inclination to stay away from others to avoid rejection and a feeling of being downwardly placed in terms of the experience of low self-esteem. In keeping with the concept of stigma power, results are consistent with the possibility that a cascade of circumstances in which stigmatized people, in seeking to avoid rejection by others, accomplish what those others want—keeping them in, down and away. Because it is new, the usefulness of the stigma power concept remains for future research to further assess. At the same time the idea that people's interests underlie their inclination to stigmatize and that these interests are often achieved in hidden misrecognizable ways is an idea that could help us understand why stigma has been so difficult to address.

Concepts described above pertaining to what stigma is, why people stigmatize, and how people use stigma to gain desired ends have grown alongside empirical studies of public conceptions or what some have called public stigma (Corrigan et al. 2004). We turn next to studies of public conceptions focusing attention on their importance as sociological phenomena and especially on the importance of assessing changes in such conceptions over time.

4.3 Public Conceptions of Mental Illnesses

One way to think about domains of public conceptions, and the most common way to do so, is to ask what determines individual differences in such conceptions and what consequences such differences might have for individual behaviors. Construed in this way, research about public conceptions is sometimes challenged when it either does not assess individual behaviors at all or predicts such behaviors with less than ideal accuracy. The lack of correspondence between attitudes and behaviors is brought to the fore and the utility of research focused on public conceptions is sharply questioned.

However, another way to reason about public conceptions that is informed a by a sociological perspective is to view them at the collective level—as indicators of cultural context. Specifically, if we could obtain an accurate and comprehensive assessment of the public conception concerning what mental illness is, what people with mental illness are like, what causes mental illnesses, what kinds of emotional reactions mental illnesses evoke, what should be done when a person develops a mental illness, how much social distance should be kept from someone with a mental illness, and what are preferred policies to address the problem of mental illness, we would have a portrait of the cultural conception of mental illness in a given place and at a particular time. It would tell us how people think and feel about mental illnesses and how such illnesses should be managed. As a context, this cultural conception becomes an external reality—something that individuals must take into account when they make decisions and enact behaviors. The idea is that individuals (e.g. people with mental illnesses, care givers, policy makers) know about cultural conceptions and shape their behaviors to some significant degree to take account of them no matter what their own knowledge, attitudes and beliefs (KABs) happen to be (see description of modified labeling theory below). In this way, cultural conceptions can have an important impact on things that matter for people with mental illnesses through mechanisms that do not involve individual attitudes influencing individual behaviors toward people with a mental illness. Consider just four ways in which cultural conceptions can affect the structural circumstances that people with mental illness encounter. First, cultural conceptions are the ways we have of thinking about the issue, about what mental illness is, what people who have mental illnesses are like, what people need, and how we should manage people who develop mental illnesses. This will influence the kind of policies and practices we conjure to address the problem, putting bounds on what we think makes sense and what we think is possible. Second, to the extent that there is a societal downward placement of mental illness in a hierarchy of importance or worthiness, structural stigma is likely to be a consequence. When studies of the prestige of medical specialties and of specific illnesses have been undertaken, psychiatry and psychiatric illness are rated low (Norredam and Album 2007). Moreover, coverage of mental illness in high-impact prestigious journals like *Lancet* is dramatically lower than one would expect given the burden of disease that mental illnesses impose (Griffiths 2010). Lower prestige and reduced coverage in major journals means less prominence that could lead to lower funding, fewer scientific discoveries and less money for good patient care. Third, cultural conceptions impose constraints on many policies and practices. For example, as treatment providers and policy makers make decisions about where to locate a new board and care home for people with serious mental illness, they are likely to include in their considerations the expected response of the neighborhoods they imagine placing the facility in. Processes like these have resulted in a clustering of board and care facilities in neighborhoods that do not have the clout to exclude such facilities, thereby creating what have been called "psychiatric ghettos" (Arboleda-Florez 2006). Fourth and finally, structural stigma is not only induced by cultural conceptions, it is also sustained by such conceptions. Imagine for example that, unlike all other illnesses, insurance policies for heart disease (instead of mental illnesses) were capped at lower levels of compensation and included higher co-pays. Despite the fact that a rationale could be conjured for such a policy, given that heart disease is influenced by behaviors people can control, such as sedentarism, fatty diets and smoking, an insurance policy disadvantaging heart disease is unimaginable at the current time. Similarly, if cultural conceptions deemed some of the disadvantages that people with mental illnesses currently endure as simply outrageous and unthinkable, pressure would be brought to bear to change them, and they would not exist.

To the extent that cultural conceptions are important, it becomes critical to understand them. Members of the Mental Health Section have taken great strides in deepening that understanding in what Pescosolido has deemed a "resurgence" of interest in this area (Pescosolido 2013). Signature accomplishments were the fielding of three mental health modules in the General Social Survey, one focused on adults views of children's mental-health disorders (Pescosolido et al. 2007) and two focused on adults' mental-health conditions that were fielded in 1996 and 2006 (Link et al. 1999; Pescosolido et al. 2010). As Pescosolido (2013) points out, these surveys have taught us a great deal and have reenergized a sociological perspective on public conceptions. Among all these accomplishments, we focus on the comparisons over time because, in our view, these are particularly revealing concerning the role of social factors over time. The reason a long-term perspective is required is that cultural conceptions change relatively slowly and it is impossible to observe such change in cross-sectional studies. Cross-sectional (or other studies with a short time frame) direct attention to the variation such studies can capture—individual differences in cultural conceptions and their associations with outcomes variables of interest. Important as such studies can be, they leave us blind to the impact of changes in levels of KABs over time and to the powerful implications such changes have for the context in which people experience mental illnesses. In keeping with this rationale, we present evidence from two studies that have enacted the same or similar methods over multiple time periods. We begin by considering a study conducted by Phelan et al. (2000) that provided evidence on changes in the stereotype of dangerousness associated with mental illness in the United States.

The Dangerousness Stereotype in the United States from 1950 to 1996. Over the period from the 1950s to the 1990s two perspectives on public attitudes were in play. On the one hand the "optimists" (Crocetti and Spiro 1974) heralded a new era in which the public was more knowledgeable and much more tolerant than it had been in the 1950s. "Pessimists" took a decidedly different and much more skeptical view, attributing any apparent positive trends to surface-level changes in knowledge about the socially desirable response to survey items (Link and Cullen 1983). There was little if any consideration of the possibility that things might have gotten worse. It was in this context that Phelan et al. undertook a study that could reflect on such changes over long periods of time.

In 1996, teams of investigators at Columbia and Indiana Universities constructed the MacArthur module of the General Social Survey (Pescosolido et al. 2010). Interested in trends over time, the team directed attention to the first nationwide U.S. study of public attitudes conducted in 1950 by Shirley Star. Unfortunately, the questions in the original study generally used language that had become dated by 1996. However, the following open-ended question was available and could be repeated, "Of course, everyone hears a good deal about physical illness and disease, but now, what about the ones we call mental or nervous illness ... When you hear someone say that a person is "mentally-ill," what does that mean to you?" In both the Star study and the MacArthur module of the 1996 survey, answers were recorded verbatim. Fortunately, every tenth interview of the original Star survey had been saved by the librarian at the National Opinion Research Center in Chicago where both studies were conducted. This allowed trained coders to reliably rate the 1950 and 1996 responses to this question with respect to whether the respondent spontaneously referred to violent behavior in describing a person with mental illness. Thereby the study allowed a rare glimpse at trends in one key stereotype in the stigma associated with mental illnesses involving psychosis. Remarkably, the analysis revealed that despite massive efforts to educate the public about mental illness and enormous advances in treatment, respondents whose descriptions indicated a person with psychosis were nearly two and a half times as likely to mention violent behavior in 1996 (31.0 %) as in 1950 (12.7 %) (Phelan et al. 2000). Whatever the reasons for this change, at the very least, it represents a discomforting fact for people with a psychotic illness seeking broader social acceptance.

Changes in Public Conceptions in the United States from 1996 to 2006. Another study of change in public conceptions used the general social survey in the United States and employed the exact same methods and measures ten years apart (Pescosolido et al. 2010). With benchmarks like the 1999 U.S. Surgeon General's report, efforts designed to reduce stigma were often predicated on assumptions that neuroscience offered the most effective tool to lower prejudice and discrimination. For example the National Alliance for the Mentally Ill's (NAMI's) "Campaign to End Discrimination" sought to improve public understanding of neurobiological bases of mental illnesses and substance abuse, facilitating treatment-seeking and lessening stigma. Over the decade between 1996 and 2006, the American public was taught about the symptoms of mental illnesses, educated about biological theories of etiology, and informed about the value of treatment to thereby underscore the basic argument that mental illnesses are diseases, no different from others. The National Stigma Study—Replication (NSS-R) which used modules from the 1996 and 2006 General Social Surveys in the United States provides evidence on the consequences of these efforts for public conceptions.

The NSS-R is a nationally representative study conducted under the umbrella of the General Social Survey that is implemented on an ongoing basis by the National Opinion Research Corporation. Individuals (N = 1,956) were interviewed face-to-face and presented with vignettes describing cases meeting DSM-IV criteria for schizophrenia, major depression or alcohol dependence. Approximately half of the respondents were interviewed in 1996, the other half in 2006, and all were randomly assigned to one vignette and then asked questions about the described person.

Results show that there were widespread increases in public acceptance of neurobiological theories about the causes of mental illnesses and significant changes in public support for treatment but no reduction in social distance or perceptions of dangerousness to self or others. Further, in both years and across all vignette conditions, holding a neurobiological conception was either unrelated to social distance and perceptions of dangerousness or was actually associated with an increase in these indicators of stigmatizing reactions (Pescosolido et al. 2010).

Again, these striking findings could not have been revealed without the trend over time, and we could not have known with any precision that the portrait of current KABs is the outcome of changes from an earlier era. Interestingly, the data provide rationales for both optimism and pessimism. On the one hand the data tell us that at least certain aspects of public conceptions are subject to change—tremendous effort was exerted to realize change and change did in fact occur in some dimensions. The public is much more likely to see mental illnesses as medical conditions and to believe that seeking help from medical and psychiatric sources is appropriate for such conditions. This change in the cultural context has been accompanied by a dramatic increase in the number of people with disorders seeking appropriate help for those disorders (Wang et al. 2005). The rational for pessimism resides in the relatively high and enduring levels of social distance and beliefs in dangerousness. There are three reasons for pessimism associated with this finding. First, a highly touted approach—advancing a neurobiological basis for mental illnesses—that was believed to be a potent factor in reducing negative attitudes failed to reduce core aspects of stigma. Second is the possibility that social distance and perceptions of danger are simply more deeply ingrained in history and the human condition and, as a consequence, much more difficult to change. Third is the possibility that social distance and stereotypes are not core concerns of the most powerful groups shaping public opinion—the medical, psychiatric and psychotherapeutic professions and pharmaceutical companies. The changes that have occurred are consistent with the interests of these groups: to be recognized on a par with other medical conditions for treating a "real" illness, to underscore the legitimacy of approaches to treatment that these groups deliver and, for the industry, an expansion of the market. Changing stereotypes and social distance are not as essential to the aims of these interest groups. People with mental illnesses who are often deeply harmed by stereotypes and rejection have great interest in these domains but less power to shape messages directed at what matters most to them.

4.3.1 Geneticization and Stigma

It certainly seems that, in the wake of the Human Genome Project and the sequencing of the human genome, genetic explanations for illness, personality, behavior, and every imaginable human characteristic are on the rise. As described above, the General Social Surveys conducted in 1996 and 2006 confirm this impression for alcohol dependence, schizophrenia, and major depression. Genetic attributions increased for all three disorders (from 61 to 71 % for schizophrenia, 51 to 64 % for major depression and 58 to 68 % for alcohol dependence) (Pescosolido et al. 2010). But what are the likely consequences of such a rise?

4.3.1.1 Theories Relating to Genetic Causal Attributions and Stigma

Attribution theory (Weiner 1986, 1995) states that the attributions people make about the cause of a personal outcome influence emotions, expectancies, and behavior toward the individual affected by the outcome. One important application of the theory has been to stigmatized behaviors (Corrigan 2000; Weiner et al. 1988).

According to the theory, attribution of low causal responsibility for a stigmatized characteristic (e.g., brain dysfunction due to accidental injury rather than illicit drug abuse) is associated with less blame and more positive emotions, that is, pity rather than anger, which in turn lead to an inclination to help the person and a disinclination to punish (Corrigan et al. 2000; Rush 1998; Weiner et al. 1988).

Because one cannot be considered to have caused one's own genetic makeup, attribution theory suggests that genetic attributions should reduce the perceived causal responsibility and, consequently, the negative emotions and behaviors associated with a stigmatized characteristic. Less sanguine predictions concerning the effect of genetic causal attributions on stigma are generated by the concept of essentialism (Rothbart and Taylor 1992) and the idea ("genetic essentialism") (Lippman 1992; Nelkin and Lindee 1995) that genetic understandings of human behavior and other characteristics increases the belief that those characteristics are an essential part of the person. In a genetic essentialist view, genes form the basis of our human and individual identities (i.e., "we are our genes") and are strongly deterministic of behavior, so that if one has genes associated with some behavior, that behavior will definitely occur and "is fixed and unchangeable" (Alper and Beckwith 1993, p. 511). A genetic essentialist viewpoint suggests that genetic characteristics are irrevocably, or at least very firmly, attached to an individual and by extension to those with whom the person shares genes. Consideration of positively valued characteristics such as beauty or intelligence make it clear that genetic essentialism is not inherently stigmatizing. However, when applied to negatively valued qualities, genetic essentialism should exacerbate stigma via its influence on several perceptions: (1) that the person is fundamentally different from others, (2) that the problem is persistent and serious, and (3) that the problem is likely to occur in other family members. These perceptions in turn should increase negative behavioral orientations such as the endorsement of reproductive restrictions and social distance, particularly "associative" (Mehta and Farina 1988) or "courtesy" stigma (Goffman 1963), in which social distance is desired from the biological relatives of the stigmatized individual.

In sum, attribution theory predicts that geneticization will reduce stigma, while the idea of genetic essentialism predicts that stigma will be exacerbated. However, different outcomes are implied by the two theories. Attribution theory predicts stigma reduction via reduced blame, anger, and punishment and increased sympathy and helping. Genetic essentialism predicts stigma magnification via increased perceptions of differentness, and—indirectly through increased perceptions of seriousness, persistence, and risk to family members—via increased social distance and reproductive restriction. Thus, it is possible that both theories are correct and operate simultaneously.

4.3.1.2 Empirical Evidence on Genetic Attributions and Stigma

We have already seen that genetic attributions increased over this period for alcohol dependence, schizophrenia and major depression but that there was no evidence that stereotypes of violence and incompetence, or the willingness to interact with people with mental illnesses changed for the better over the period between the studies (Pescosolido et al. 2010). This evidence challenges the idea that stigma will dissipate when the public is moved toward more medical and genetic views of mental illnesses. A review of additional evidence, much of it experimental, was conducted by Phelan and Link (2012). They located 17 studies that examined the association between genetic attributions and stigma-related outcomes for a variety of stigmatized characteristics (Angermeyer et al. 2003; Bennett et al. 2008; Boyle et al. 2009; Dietrich et al. 2004; Eker 1985; Feldman and Crandall 2007; Jorm and Griffiths 2008; Magliano et al. 2004; Martin et al. 2000; Menec and Perry 1998; Phelan 2002, 2005; Phelan et al. 2006; Piskur and Degelman 1992; Schnittker 2008; Teachman et al. 2003). These focused primarily on mental illnesses (N = 12) and usually specifically on schizophrenia (N = 11) and/or major depression (N = 9). The most commonly studied stigma-related outcome was social distance (N = 11). Other outcomes included blame, perceived dangerousness, unpredictability and incompetence, emotions of anger and sympathy, and intentions to help, punish or restrict reproduction. Nine of the studies employed experimental designs, randomly assigning research participants to be exposed to different causal statements. The eight non-experimental studies assessed participants' causal beliefs and stigmatizing attitudes and measured the relationship between the two. The studies more often indicate a stigmatizing effect of genetic attributions than a de-stigmatizing effect, but the findings are far from consistent. Nineteen significant positive associations (P < 0.05) between genetic explanations and stigma, eight significant negative associations (P < 0.05), and twenty-eight non-significant associations were reported in these 17 studies. Importantly, these stigmatizing effects varied by outcome in ways that speak to the two theories (attribution and essentialism) that have been applied to understand them.

First, when outcomes specified by attribution theory—blame, anger, punishment, pity and willingness to help—were examined, 13 associations were found. Four were significant in a direction consistent with attribution theory whereas in the other nine no significant associations were uncovered. Second, when outcomes specified by the theory of genetic essentialism—seriousness, persistence, differentness and the spread of stigma to genetically related individuals—12 were found. Six associations concerned perceived seriousness and persistence and four of these were significant in the direction predicted by essentialist predictions. Genetic attribution was not significantly related to persistence in another instance and was not associated with perceived differentness in the one case where differentness was examined. Four other associations relevant to essentialist predictions concerned associative stigma measured in terms of desired social distance from the relative of a person who was described as having a genetically caused disorder. In all four instances significant associations were found.

In sum, the preponderance of results suggested stigmatizing rather than de-stigmatizing effects of genetic attributions, but this pattern was by no means strong or dramatic. There were a considerable number of non-significant associations as well as a number of instances in which genetic attribution was associated with less stigma. Focusing on outcomes related to the two theoretical perspectives with specific relevance to genetic explanations for stigmatized characteristics, the number of relevant findings is small, but somewhat more consistent. Although we still find non-significant associations, all statistically significant findings are in the predicted direction. Clearly, the number of findings reviewed by Phelan and Link is too small to draw firm conclusions; nevertheless they are suggestive that genetic attributions may have opposite effects on stigma through the dual pathways of reducing blame and increasing genetic essentialism.

More generally, and in keeping with the GSS results concerning population change, these results tell us that there is no easy fix to public stigma. We cannot just convince the public that mental illnesses are genetically based biological illnesses and expect issues of stigma to be resolved.

4.4 Personal Consequences of Stigma for People with Mental Illnesses

Interest in how people with mental illnesses are affected by stigma and how they seek to cope with or resist such stigmatization has been a central concern for members of the Section on the Sociology of Mental Health. We begin our consideration of these issues by focusing attention on modified labeling theory (Link 1982, 1987; Link et al. 1989) and evidence that has accumulated about that theory. It is an auspicious place to start because it links public conceptions (the focus of the last section) with personal consequences (the focus of this section).

Modified Labeling Theory. In the 1980s Link and his colleagues developed a "modified" labeling theory that derived insights from the original labeling theory, but stepped away from the claim that labeling is a direct cause of mental illness (Link 1982, 1987; Link et al. 1989). Instead the theory postulated a process through which labeling and stigma jeopardize the life circumstances of people with mental illnesses, harming their employment chances, social networks, and self-esteem. By creating disadvantage in these domains and others like them, people who have experienced mental illness labels are put at greater risk of the prolongation or reoccurrence of mental illness. The modified labeling theory also provided an explanation as to how labeling and stigma might produce these effects and how key concepts and measures could be used in testing the explanation with empirical evidence.

The theory begins with the observation that people develop conceptions of mental illness early in life as part of socialization (Angermeyer and Matschinger 1996; Scheff 1966; Wahl 1995). Once in place, people's conceptions become a lay theory about what it means to have a mental illness (Angermeyer and Matschinger 1994; Furnham and Bower 1992). People form expectations as to whether most people will reject an individual with mental illness as a friend, employee, neighbor, or intimate partner and whether most people will devalue a person with mental illness as less trustworthy, intelligent, and competent. These beliefs have an especially poignant relevance for a person who develops a serious mental illness, because the possibility of devaluation and discrimination becomes personally relevant. If one believes that others will devalue and reject people with mental illness, one must now fear that this rejection will apply personally. The person may wonder, "Will others look down on me, reject me, simply because I have been identified as having a mental illness?" Then, to the extent that it becomes a part of a person's worldview, that perception can have serious negative consequences that affect self-confidence, social relationships, employment and other life-domains.

To test this explanation, Link (1987) constructed a 12-item scale measuring the extent to which a person believes that people who have been labeled by treatment contact will be devalued and discriminated against. Respondents are asked the extent to which they agree or disagree with statements indicating that most people devalue current or former psychiatric patients by seeing them as failures, as less intelligent than other persons, or as individuals whose opinions need not be taken seriously. The scale also includes items that assess perceived discrimination by most people in jobs, friendships, and romantic relationships. The scale was administered to people with mental illnesses and to community residents from the same general area of New York City in a case-control study of major depression and schizophrenia. Link (1987) showed that the degree to which a person expects to be rejected is associated with demoralization, income loss, and unemployment. This association occurs in individuals labeled mentally ill but not in unlabeled individuals, thereby supporting the idea that labeling activates beliefs that lead to negative consequences.

Link et al. (1989) extended the forgoing reasoning in two ways. First they brought into the analysis empirical measures of coping orientations of secrecy (concealing a history of treatment), withdrawal (avoiding potentially threatening situations), and education (attempting to teach others in order to forestall the negative effects of stereotypes). Consistent with the idea that the stigma associated with mental illness creates expectations of rejection, they showed that people with mental illnesses tend to endorse these strategies as a means of protecting themselves. Second, the researchers extended the analysis to a consideration of the effects of these processes on social network ties. They found that people who fear rejection most and who endorse the strategy of withdrawal have insular support networks consisting mainly of household members.

Aspects of the theory have since been tested with a broader range of outcomes, in different samples, by different investigators, and often using longitudinal data. These studies generally showed that the perceived devaluation-discrimination measure is associated with outcome variables including quality of life (Rosenfield 1997), self-esteem (Link et al. 2001, 2008; Livingston and Boyd 2010; Wright et al. 2000), social networks (Link et al. 1989; Perlick et al. 2001) depressive symptoms (Link et al. 1997; Perlick et al. 2007), treatment adherence (Sirey et al. 2001) and treatment discontinuation (Sirey et al. 2001). But one particular aspect of the theory, the idea that cultural conceptions (perceived devaluation and discrimination) have effects on outcome variables in labeled persons but not in unlabeled ones, has not been as thoroughly tested in subsequent research. One study that did do so was undertaken by Kroska and Harkness (2006) using samples of psychiatric hospital patients and community residents in Indianapolis. This study operationalized cultural conceptions in a completely different way than Link and his colleagues did. Patients and community residents were asked to evaluate the concept "mentally ill person" using a seven-point semantic differential scale with opposing adjectives such as "good/bad," "useful/useless," and "powerless/powerful." Respondents also rated the concept "myself as I really am" and "myself as others see me" with the same adjective pairings. The researchers' modified labeling theory hypothesis was that associations between ratings of the concept "mentally ill person" and "myself as I really am" and "myself as others see me" concepts would be stronger in the labeled group (where a mental illness label is potentially personally relevant) than in the unlabeled group (where it is not personally relevant). Their results were generally consistent with this prediction, providing additional support for this key prediction of modified labeling theory.

Labeling as a "Package Deal." Evidence from modified labeling theory and other approaches to labeling, stereotyping, and rejection strongly suggest that negative consequences associated with labeling are experienced by many people. At the same time, evidence from a voluminous body of research indicates that a variety of psychotherapies and drug therapies can be helpful in treating many mental illnesses. Given this, existing data simply do not justify a continued debate concerning whether the effects of labeling are positive or negative—clearly they are both. Rosenfield (1997) was the first to bring this point to light in a single study. She examined the effects of both treatment services and stigma in the context of a model program for people with severe mental illnesses. She showed that both the receipt of services (specific interventions that some people in the program receive and others do not) and stigma (Link's 1987 measure of perceived devaluation and discrimination) are related—in opposite directions—to multiple dimensions of a quality of life measure. Receipt of services had positive effects on dimensions of quality of life, such as living arrangements, family relations, financial situation, safety, and health, whereas stigma had equally strong negative effects on such dimensions.

A second study that explores the idea of joint effects in opposite directions is one by Link et al. (1997). In a longitudinal study, men who were dually diagnosed with mental disorder and substance abuse were followed from entry into treatment (when they were highly symptomatic and addicted to substances) to a follow-up point one year later (when they were far less symptomatic and largely drug- and alcohol-free). Despite these dramatic benefits, the results also showed that perceptions of devaluation and discrimination and reported experiences of discrimination continued to affect the men's level of depressive symptoms. Similar results, showing evidence of improvement in symptoms with treatment but enduring effects of stigma on self-esteem, were reported in a recent study by Link et al. (2008). The effects of stigma and discrimination endure and are apparently unaffected by any benefits of treatment.

Thus the evidence indicates a bundling of labeling effects that are currently joined in a kind of "package deal." People seeking mental health treatment navigate this deal in one way or another. Sometimes they do so in ways that mental health professionals think they should not, such as avoiding treatment, denying their illness, or ending treatment earlier than their treatment team thinks they should. A kind of collective finger-wagging ensues that at times shifts from admonitions and warnings to using the "leverage" of housing or financial benefits to ensure treatment compliance (Monahan et al. 2001). If leverage fails, more direct forms of coercion are also possible such as involuntary inpatient commitment or the ascendant "outpatient commitment"(Hiday 2003). Of course, there is an intense debate about the utility and effectiveness of leverage and coercion, with some believing that these practices are necessary (Torrey and Zdanowicz 2001) and others seeing them as counterproductive (Pollack 2004). What a sociological perspective adds to this debate is evidence that there is indeed a package deal and that people face real choices and real dilemmas as they navigate its parameters. It also suggests that the ingenuity invested in constructing strategies to leverage compliance or to coerce it needs to be complemented or replaced by efforts that really change the balance of the package deal to one that delivers more benefit and less stigma. When that happens, more people will choose treatment, and less leveraging and coercion will be required. Mental health sociologists can help by continuing to unpack the package deal so that its existence is more widely acknowledged and our understanding of the mechanisms that undergird it more complete. Recent research by mental health sociologists is engaged in precisely these issues. For example, Markowitz and Angell (2011) elaborated on the modified labeling theory to probe more deeply into the mechanisms involved by including the reflected appraisals of family members in their empirical analysis. Lucas and Phelan (2012) conducted experimental work integrating paradigms from the expectation-states tradition in sociology (Berger et al. 1972) with work in psychology on the sources of stigma in interaction processes to investigate whether and to what extent a mental illness label reduces influence in interactions and engenders behavioral social distance. Identifying sources, probing mechanisms, and evaluating novel attempts to respond to stigma will deepen our understanding and enable us to address the stigma processes that affect people with mental illnesses.

4.4.1 Stigma Coping and Stigma Resistance

Individually-Based Stigma Coping Responses. The idea that people who are stigmatized actively respond to their situation has been a central element of theories about stigma ever since the concept emerged as a critical social scientific idea in the 1960s. It is, for example, a key component of classic labeling theory's concept of "secondary deviance" as something brought on by "defense, attack, or adaptation" to the overt or covert problems produced by societal reactions to "primary deviance" (Lemert 1967, p. 17). And of course Goffman's (1963) essay is all about the active "management" of stigma both by those who are the object of stigma and by those who do the stigmatizing. This active response to stigma is carried forward by Link et al. (1989, 1991, 2002) in the empirical elaboration of modified labeling theory through the conceptualization and measurement of stigma coping orientations. In earlier work, coping orientations of "secrecy" (concealing labeling information) "education" (providing information to counter stereotypes) and "withdrawal" (avoiding potentially rejecting situations) were measured and assessed (Link et al. 1989, 1991) followed by the addition of coping orientations of "challenging" and "distancing" (Link et al. 2002). Challenging is the active confrontation of stigmatizing behavior. For example, one might challenge by pointing out stigmatizing behavior when it occurs and by indicating that one disagrees with the content of stigmatizing statements or disapproves of stigmatizing behaviors. Distancing is a cognitive separation of the potentially stigmatized person from the stigmatized group. In distancing, one dodges the stereotype that others might apply or that one might apply to oneself by essentially saying—"I am not like them!" "Your stereotypes of them are misapplied to me."

But if both classic and modified labeling theories have emphasized the active response of the stigmatized, what are the consequences of these efforts according to these research traditions? Are individually-based efforts to cope or resist effective? The concept of secondary deviance suggests not—at least not always. The responses of "defense, attack or adaptation" by the stigmatized induce additional "secondary" deviance that further sets the person apart (Lemert 1967). And, when Link et al. (1991) assessed the coping orientations of secrecy, education and withdrawal, they found no evidence that these approaches buffered people with mental illnesses from untoward consequences, but did find some evidence that these orientations actually exacerbated these consequences. They conclude that individual coping orientations are unlikely to be effective because they do not deal with the fundamental problem of deeply embedded cultural conceptions and stereotypes. According to Link et al. (1991), the best solutions are ones that change societal conceptions or involve the collective action of people with mental illnesses that change power differentials.

More recently, Thoits (2011) developed new concepts and theory suggesting the possibility of "stigma resistance" at the individual level particularly as it might protect the self-esteem of people with mental illnesses. Thoits points to what she calls a moderate association between perceived or experienced stigma and self-esteem and infers that a less than perfect association means that some people effectively counteract the effects of stigma on self-esteem. Thoits identifies two forms of resistance: "deflecting, impeding or refusing to yield to the penetration of a harmful force or influence" and "challenging, confronting, or fighting a harmful force or influence" (Thoits 2011, p. 11). In "deflecting," a person responds to mental illness and associated stereotypes by concluding "that's not me," "that is only a small unimportant part of me," or that the designation "mentally ill" does not apply to me because my problems are something different than mental illness. According to Thoits (2011, p. 14), deflecting strategies offer the possibility to "dramatically reduce, if not eliminate, potential threats to self-regard." "Challenging" as described by Thoits (2011) differs from deflecting in that it involves an effort to change other people's beliefs or behaviors. A person can challenge by (1) behaving in ways that contradict stereotypes, (2) educating others to move them away from stereotyped views, (3) confronting people who express prejudicial sentiments and behave in discriminatory ways, or (4) engaging in advocacy and activism.

Whether, to what extent and under what conditions stigma resistance can protect self regard or other potential consequences of stigma is an empirical question that has not been fully resolved. Our conjecture is that individually based efforts will generally fail. We base this in part on Link et al.'s (1991) study suggesting that at least three individually-based coping approaches (secrecy, withdrawal and education) were not effective in reducing distress or counteracting negative consequences for employment for people with mental illnesses. Additionally, although there is something alluring about the idea that the stigmatized can fight back or cognitively manipulate their orientation to stigmatizing circumstances, one must keep in mind that stigmatizers are actively pursuing their own interests at the same time. To the extent that stigmatizers have an interest in keeping people, down, in or away we can expect them to counter the efforts of stigmatized groups to resist with the exercise of power. Foucault's famous aphorism "Where there is power there is resistance" can be turned around to read "where there is resistance there is power." Agency is operative for both the stigmatized and the stigmatizer and it is likely that the ultimate outcome will depend on the relative power of the two groups. This leads to our pessimism about individually-based coping or resistance—the actions of single individuals are very unlikely to change the power difference between stigmatized and stigmatizing groups.

Group-based Resistance—Social Movements. We are much more optimistic about the long-term effectiveness of group-based resistance. One reason is that we can point to some social movements that have been at least partially successful such as the civil rights movement and the gay and lesbian liberation movement. Another reason is that sustained collective action over long periods of time affects a mechanism we believe is critical to the successful production of stigma—it alters the balance of power between stigmatizing and stigmatized groups thereby altering the capacity of the stigmatizing group to exert their desire to keep people down, in or away. In the long run it may even change the stigmatizers' inclination to keep people down, in or away. This is not to say that collective social action proceeds in a linear fashion toward success. Instead collective action proceeds in fits and starts, sometimes gaining ground, sometimes losing it and sometimes failing altogether. But social movements usually aim to directly resist the power of the stigmatizing groups, thereby seeking changes that can be sustained over time. Interestingly, research has shown just how important sociological processes are in such social movements (Jasper 2011). For example, social movements of stigmatized groups often seek a shift in identity from shame to pride, set in place interaction rituals that sustain commitment, manipulate "moral shocks" to recruit new members and keep old ones engaged by highlighting or otherwise enhancing the emotional impact of events (Jasper 2011). In sum, sociological processes are critical to understanding stigma coping and resistance, and both individually-based and group-based resistance should be studied from a sociological perspective. What we expect is that individually-based efforts will be less effective in resisting stigma than group-based social movements and that this will be especially true if one adopts a long-term perspective.

4.4.2 The Future

This chapter provided examples of sociologically inspired efforts to conceptualize and understand mental illness stigma. A definition of stigma that includes multiple components and that is attentive to the power differences between stigmatizers and the stigmatized was one such example. Another was the sociologically informed inquiry into why people stigmatize with its focus on the interests stigmatizers have in keeping people down, in or away. Viewed from this vantage point stigma is form of power, a way that people achieve desired outcomes. The chapter also provided examples of research concerning public conceptions, how such conceptions are distinctly sociological and how much progress has been made in recent years in understanding them. Finally, the chapter provided an example in the form of modified labeling theory of a sociological approach to understanding how stigma harms people with mental illnesses and also evidence about how people seek to side step or resist the impact of stigma on their lives. In light of this work it seems fair to say that substantial progress has been made in the sociological understanding of mental illness stigma. At the same time, it is also true that large gaps in understanding remain. In particular, there is much to be done in terms of filling out the promise of some of the concepts and theories that have already been introduced and, of course, new concepts and understandings are likely to emerge in the time ahead. But we end with one recommendation for the future and that is the development of a sociologically informed approach to stigma change.

Sociologists are trained to be adept observers who use their sociological imagination to understand social processes. Of course this kind of understanding carries the capacity to create change, especially to the extent that it reveals processes that might otherwise be hidden. Whereas 50 years ago the word stigma was rarely used, today it is widely employed to bring to light the predicaments faced by people experiencing a wide variety of circumstances. It is difficult to quantify the effect of such a transformation but to the extent that people can identify the processes that trouble them we presume they will be more able to challenge and perhaps change them. Still, if stigma processes are deeply set in sociological phenomena, it would seem that sociologists could play an active role in conjuring ways to change stigma processes. This is rare. Elaine Cummings, a sociologist, collaborated with her husband John Cummings, a psychiatrist, in an effort to change attitudes in a town in Saskatchewan, Canada in the early 1950s. The failed attempt was published in the now classic and extremely instructive book, *Closed Ranks* (1957). But since that undertaking, sociologists have only rarely engaged in efforts to change mental illness stigma. We believe that such an undertaking represents a strong challenge for the future mental health sociology—to lay out a sociologically informed strategy and to suggest lynch-pin intervention approaches that could move that strategy forward.

References

Alper, J. S., & Beckwith, J. (1993). Genetic fatalism and social policy: The implications of behavior genetics research. *The Yale Journal of Biology and Medicine, 66*(6), 511–524.
Angermeyer, M. C., & Matschinger, H. (1994). Lay beliefs about schizophrenic disorder: The results of a population survey in Germany. *Acta Psychiatrica Scandinavica Supplementum, 382*, 39–45.
Angermeyer, M. C., & Matschinger, H. (1996). Public attitude towards psychiatric treatment. *Psychiatrica Scandinavica, 94*, 326–336.
Angermeyer, M. C., Matschinger, H., & Corrigan, P. W. (2003). Familiarity with mental illness and social distance from people with schizophrenia and major depression: Testing a model using data from a representative population survey. *Schizophrenia Research, 69*, 175–182.
Arboleda-Florez, J. (2006). Forensic psychiatry: contemporary scope, challenges and controversies. *World Psychiatry, 5*(2), 87–91.
Bennett, L., Thirlaway, K., & Murray, A. J. (2008). The stigmatising implications of presenting schizophrenia as a genetic disease. *Journal of Genetic Counseling, 17*(6), 550–559.
Berger, J., Bernard, P. C., & Zelditch, J. M. (1972). Status characteristics and social interaction. *American Sociological Review, 37*, 241–255.
Bourdieu, P. (1987). What makes a social class? On the theoretical and practical existence of groups. *Berkeley Journal of Sociology, 32*, 1–18.
Bourdieu, P. (1990). *The logic of practice*. Stanford: Stanford University Press.
Boyle, M. P., Blood, G. W., & Blood, I. M. (2009). Effects of perceived causality on perceptions of persons who stutter. *Journal of Fluency Disorders, 34*(3), 201–218.
Corrigan, P. W. (2000). Mental health stigma as social attribution: Implications for research methods and attitude change. *Clinical Psychology: Science and Practice, 7*, 48–67.
Corrigan, P. W., Markowitz, F. E., & Watson, A. C. (2004). Structural levels of mental illness stigma and discrimination. *Schizophrenia Bulletin, 30*(3), 481–491.
Corrigan, P. W., River, L. P., Lundin, R. K., Wasowski, K. U., Campion, J., Mathisen, J., et al. (2000). Stigmatizing attributions about mental illness. *Journal of Community Psychology, 28*, 91–103.
Crocetti, G., & Spiro, H. (1974). *Contemporary attitudes towards mental illness*. Pittsburgh, PA: University of Pittsburgh Press.
Cumming, E., & Cumming, J. (1957). *Closed ranks: An experiment in mental health education*. Cambridge, Massachusetts: Harvard University Press.
Dietrich, S., Beck, M., Bujantugs, B., Kenzine, D., Matschinger, H., & Angermeyer, M. C. (2004). The relationship between public causal beliefs and social distance toward mentally ill people. *Australian and New Zealand Journal of Psychiatry, 38*(5), 348–354.
Eker, D. (1985). Effect of type of cause on attitudes toward mental illness and relationships between the attitudes. *International Journal of Social Psychiatry, 31*(4), 243–251.
Erikson, K. T. (1966). *Wayward puritan: A study in the sociology of deviance*. New York: Wiley.
Feagin, J. R. (2009). *The white racial frame: Centuries of racial framing and counter-framing*. New York: Routledge.
Feldman, D. B., & Crandall, C. S. (2007). Dimensions of mental illness stigma: What about mental illness causes social rejection? *Journal of Social and Clinical Psychology, 26*(2), 137–154.
Fine, M., & Asche, A. (1988). Disability beyond stigma: Social interaction, discrimination an activism. *Journal of Social Issues, 44*, 3–22.
Furnham, A., & Bower, P. (1992). A comparison of academic and lay theories of schizophrenia. *British Journal of Psychiatry, 161*, 201–210.
Goffman, E. (1961). *Asylums*. Garden City, NY: Doubleday.
Goffman, E. (1963). *Stigma: Notes on the management of spoiled identity*. New York: Simon & Schuster.
Gove, W. R. (1975). *The labeling of deviance: Evaluating a perspective*. New York: Sage.
Gove, W. R. (1982). The current status of the labeling theory of mental illness. In W. R. Gove (Ed.), *Deviance and mental Illness* (pp. 273–300). Beverly Hills, CA: Sage.

Griffiths, K. (2010, June 10). *Unraveling the stigma of depression*. Paper presented at the meetings of the Academy of Eating Disorders, Salzburg, Germany.

Hiday, V. A. (2003). Outpatient commitment: The state of empirical research on its outcomes. *Psychology, Public Policy, and Law, 9*(1–2), 8–32.

Horwitz, A., & Wakefield, J. (2007). *The loss of sadness*. New York: Oxford University Press.

Jasper, J. M. (2011). Emotions and social movements: Twenty years of theory and research. *Annual Review of Sociology, 37*(14), 285–303.

Jones, E. A., Farina, A., Hastorf, A., Markus, H., Miller, D. T., & Scott, R. (1984). *Social stigma: The psychology of marked relationships*. New York: Freeman.

Jorm, A. F., & Griffiths, K. M. (2008). The public's stigmatizing attitudes towards people with mental disorders: How important are biomedical conceptualizations? *Acta Psychiatrica Scandinavica, 118*(4), 315–321. doi:10.1111/j.1600-0447.2008.01251.x.

Kroska, A., & Harkness, S. K. (2006). Stigma sentiments and self-meanings: Exploring the modified labeling theory of mental illness. *Social Psychology Quarterly, 69*, 325–348.

Kurzban, R., & Leary, M. R. (2001). Evolutionary origins of stigmatization: The functions of social exclusion. *Psychological Bulletin, 127*(2), 187–208.

Lemert, E. (1967). *Human deviance, social problems, and social control*. Englewood Cliffs, NJ: Prentice Hall.

Link, B., Castille, D. M., & Stuber, J. (2008). Stigma and coercion in the context of outpatient treatment for people with mental illnesses. *Social Science and Medicine, 67*(3), 409–419.

Link, B. G. (1982). Mental patient status, work, and income: An examination of the effects of a psychiatric label. *American Sociological Review, 47*(2), 202–215.

Link, B. G. (1987). Understanding labeling effects in the area of mental disorders: An assessment of the effects of expectations of rejection. *American Sociological Review, 52*, 96–112.

Link, B. G., & Cullen, F. T. (1983). Reconsidering the social rejection of ex-mental patients: Levels of attitudinal response. *American Journal of Community Psychology, 11*(3), 261–273.

Link, B. G., Cullen, F. T., Struening, E., Shrout, P., & Dohrenwend, B. P. (1989). A modified labeling theory approach in the area of mental disorders: An empirical assessment. *American Sociological Review, 54*, 400–423.

Link, B. G., Mirotznik, J., & Cullen, F. T. (1991). The effectiveness of stigma coping orientations: Can negative consequences of mental illness labeling be avoided? *Journal of Health and Social Behavior, 32*, 302–320.

Link, B. G., & Phelan, J. C. (2001). Conceptualizing stigma. *Annual Review of Sociology, 27*, 363–385.

Link, B. G., & Phelan, J. C. (2014). Stigma power. *Social Science & Medicine, 103*, 24–32.

Link, B. G., Phelan, J. C., Bresnahan, M., Stueve, A., & Pescosolido, B. A. (1999). Public conceptions of mental illness: Labels, causes, dangerousness, and social distance. *American Journal Public Health, 89*(9), 1328–1333.

Link, B. G., Struening, E. L., Neese-Todd, S., Asmussen, S., & Phelan, J. C. (2001). Stigma as a barrier to recovery: The consequences of stigma for the self-esteem of people with mental illnesses. *Psychiatric Services (Washington, D.C.), 52*(12), 1621–1626.

Link, B. G., Struening, E. L., Neese-Todd, S., Asmussen, S., & Phelan, J. C. (2002). On describing and seeking to change the experience of stigma. *Psychiatric Rehabilitation Skills, 6*, 201–231.

Link, B. G., Struening, E. L., Rahav, M., Phelan, J. C., & Nuttbrock, L. (1997). On stigma and its consequences: Evidence from a longitudinal study of men with dual diagnoses of mental illness and substance abuse. *Journal of Health and Social Behavior, 38*(2), 177–190.

Link, B. G., Yang, L. H., Phelan, J. C., & Collins, P. Y. (2004). Measuring mental illness stigma. *Schizophrenia Bulletin, 30*(3), 511–541.

Lippman, A. (1992). Led (astray) by genetic maps: The cartography of the human genome and healthcare. *Social Science and Medicine, 35*(12), 1469–1476.

Livingston, J. D., & Boyd, J. E. (2010). Correlates and consequences of internalized stigma for people living with mental illness: A systematic review and meta-analysis. *Social Science and Medicine, 71*, 2150–2161.

Lucas, J., & Phelan, J. C. (2012). Status and stigma: The interrelation of two theoretical perspectives. *Social Psychology Quarterly, 75*, 310–333.
Magliano, L., Fiorillo, A., Guarneri, M., Marasco, C., De Rosa, C., & Malangone, C. (2004). Prescription of psychotropic drugs to patients with schizophrenia : An Italian national survey. *European Journal of Clinical Pharmacology, 60*(7), 513–522.
Major, B., & O'Brien, L. T. (2005). The social psychology of stigma. *Annual Review of Psychology, 56*, 393–421.
Markowitz, F. E., Angell, B., & Greenberg, J. S. (2011). Stigma, reflected appraisals and recovery outcomes in mental illness. *Social Psychology Quarterly, 74*, 144–165.
Martin, J., Pescosolido, B., & Tuch, S. (2000). Of fear and loathing: The role of "disturbing behavior," labels, and causal attributions in shaping public attitudes toward people with mental illness. *Journal of Health and Social Behavior, 41*, 208–223.
Mehta, S., & Farina, A. (1988). Associative stigma: Perceptions of the difficulties of college-aged children of stigmatized fathers. *Journal of Social Clinical Psychology, 7*, 192–202.
Menec, V. H., & Perry, R. P. (1998). Reactions to stigmas among Canadian students: Testing attribution-affect-help judgement model. *Journal of Social Psychology, 138*, 443–453.
Monahan, J., Bonnie, R. J., Appelbaum, P. S., Hyde, P. S., Steadman, H. J., & Swartz, M. S. (2001). Mandated community treatment: Beyond outpatient commitment. *Psychiatric Services (Washington, D.C.), 52*(9), 1198–1205.
Morone, J. A. (1997). Enemies of the people: The moral dimension to public health. *Journal of Health Politics, Policy and Law, 22*, 993–1020.
Nelkin, D., & Lindee, M. S. (1995). *The DNA mystique: The gene as a cultural icon.* New York: Freeman.
Norredam, M., & Album, D. (2007). Prestige and its significance for medical specialties and diseases. *Scandinavian Journal of Public Health, 35*, 655–661.
Oliver, M. (1992). *The politics of disablement.* Basingstoke: MacMillian.
Perlick, D. A., Rosenheck, R. A., Clarkin, J. F., Sirey, J. A., Salahi, J., Struening, E. L., et al. (2001). Stigma as a barrier to recovery: Adverse effects of perceived stigma on social adaptation of persons diagnosed with bipolar affective disorder. *Psychiatric Services (Washington, D.C.), 52*(12), 1627–1632.
Perlick, D. A., Rosenheck, R. A., Miklowitz, D. J., Chessick, C., Wolff, N., Kaczynski, R., & Group, S.-B. F. E. C. S. (2007). Prevalence and correlates of burden among caregivers of patients with bipolar disorder enrolled in the Systematic Treatment Enhancement Program for Bipolar Disorder. *Bipolar Disord, 9*(3), 262–273.
Parker, R., & Aggleton, P. (2003). HIV and AIDS-related stigma and discrimination: A conceptual framework and implications for action. *Social Science and Medicine, 57*, 13–24.
Pescosolido, B. A. (2013). The public stigma of mental illness: What do we think; what do we know what can we prove? *Journal of Health and Social Behavior, 54*(1), 1–21.
Pescosolido, B. A., Fettes, D. L., Martin, J. K., Monahan, J., & McLeod, J. D. (2007). Perceived dangerousness of children with mental health problems and support for coerced treatment. *Psychiatric Services (Washington, D. C.), 58*(5), 619–625. doi:10.1176/appi.ps.58.5.619.
Pescosolido, B. A., Martin, J. K., Long, J. S., Medina, T. R., Phelan, J. C., & Link, B. G. (2010). "A disease like any other"? A decade of change in public reactions to schizophrenia, depression, and alcohol dependence. *American Journal of Psychiatry, 167*(11), 1321–1330.
Phelan, J. C. (2002). Genetic bases of mental illness—a cure for stigma? [review]. *Trends in Neurosciences, 25*(8), 430–431.
Phelan, J. C. (2005). Geneticization of deviant behavior: Consequences for stigma the case of mental illness. *Journal of Health and Behavioral Science, 46*, 307–322.
Phelan, J.C. & Link B. G. (2012). Genetics, addiction and stigma. In A. R. Chapman (Ed.), *Genetic research on addiction: Ethics, law and public health* (pp. 174–194). New York: Cambridge.
Phelan, J. C., Link, B. G., & Dovidio, J. F. (2008). Stigma and prejudice: One animal or two? *Social Science and Medicine, 67*(3), 358–367. doi:10.1016/j.socscimed.2008.03.022.

Phelan, J. C., Link, B. G., Stueve, A., & Pescosolido, B. A. (2000). Public conceptions of mental illness in 1950 and 1996: What is mental illness and is it to be feared? *Journal of Health and Social Behavior, 41*, 188–207.

Phelan, J. C., Yang, L. H., & Cruz-Rojas, R. (2006). Effects of attributing serious mental illnesses to genetic causes on orientations to treatment. *Psychiatric Services (Washington, D. C.), 57*(3), 382–387.

Piskur, J., & Degelman, D. (1992). Effect of reading a summary of research about biological bases of homosexual orientation on attitudes toward homosexuals. *Psychological Reports, 71*(3 Pt 2), 1219–1225.

Pollack, D. A. (2004). *Moving from coercion to collaboration in mental health services.* Rockville, MD: Center for Mental Health Services, Substance Abuse and Mental Health Services Administration.

Rabkin, J. (1984). Determinants of public attitudes about mental illness: Summary of the research literature. *Attitudes Toward the Mentally Ill: Research Perspectives, 10*, 15–26.

Rosenfield, S. (1997). Labeling mental illness: The effects of received services and perceived stigma on life satisfaction. *American Sociological Review, 62*, 660–672.

Rothbart, M., & Taylor, M. (1992). Category labels and social reality: Do we view social categories as natural kinds? In G. R. S. Semin & K. Fiedler (Eds.), *Language, interaction and social cognition* (pp. 11–36). Newbury Park, CA: Sage.

Rush, L. L. (1998). Affective reactions to multiple stigmas. *Journal of Social Psychology, 138*, 421–430.

Scheff, T. J. (1966). *Being mentally ill: A sociological theory.* Chicago: Oxford.

Schnittker, J. (2008). An uncertain revolution: Why the rise of a genetic model of mental illness has not increased tolerance. *Social Science and Medicine, 67*(9), 1370–1381.

Schwartz, C. G. (1956). The stigma of mental illness. *Journal of Rehabilitation, 22*, 7–29.

Sirey, J. A., Bruce, M. L., Alexopoulos, G. S., Perlick, D. A., Friedman, S. J., & Meyers, B. S. (2001). Stigma as a barrier to recovery: Perceived stigma and patient-rated severity of illness as predictors of antidepressant drug adherence. *Psychiatric Services, 52*, 1615–1620.

Teachman, B. A., Gapinski, K. D., Brownell, K. D., Rawlins, M., & Jeyaram, S. (2003). Demonstrations of implicit anti-fat bias: The impact of providing causal information and evoking empathy. *Health Psychology, 22*(1), 68–78.

Thoits, P. A. (1985). Self-labeling processes in mental illness: The role of emotional deviance. *American Journal of Sociology, 92*, 221–249.

Thoits, P. A. (2011). Resisting the stigma of mental illness. *Social Psychology Quarterly, 74*, 6–28.

Torrey, E. F., & Zdanowicz, M. (2001). Outpatient commitment: What, why, and for whom. *Psychiatric Services (Washington, D. C.), 52*(3), 337–341.

Wahl, O. F. (1995). *Media madness: Public images of mental illness.* New Brunswick, NJ: Rutgers University Press.

Wang, P. S., Lane, M., Olfson, M., Pincus, H. A., Wells, K. B., & Kessler, R. C. (2005). Twelve-month use of mental health services in the United States: Results from the National Comorbidity Survey Replication. *Archives of General Psychiatry, 62*(6), 629–640.

Weiner, B. (1986). *Attributional theory of motivation and emotion.* New York: Springer.

Weiner, B. (1995). *Judgements of responsibility: A foundation for a theory of social conduct.* New York: Guilford Press.

Weiner, B., Perry, R. P., & Magnusson, J. (1988). An attributional analysis of reactions to stigmas. *Journal of Personality and Social Psychology, 55*(5), 738–748.

Wright, E. R., Gonfrein, W. P., & Owens, T. J. (2000). Deinstitutionalization, social rejection, and the self-esteem of former mental patients. *Journal of Health and Social Behavior, 41*, 68–90.

Yang, L. H., Kleinman, A., Link, B. G., Phelan, J. C., Lee, S., & Good, B. (2007). Culture and stigma: Adding moral experience to stigma theory. *Social Science and Medicine, 64*(7), 1524–1535.

Chapter 5
The Neighborhood and Mental Life: Past, Present, and Future Sociological Directions in Studying Community Context and Mental Health

Richard M. Carpiano

How do the social and physical environments of neighborhoods and other local places matter for the mental health and well-being of their residents? Even a casual scan of article titles within the leading medical sociology journals over the past 20 years will reveal that there has been an intense interest in this complex and multifaceted research question. This question is not simply of interest to academics. It has important implications for practice and policy, in terms of primary and secondary prevention as well as service provision. Like most areas of sociological inquiry, research on place and mental health is not a new area of research. This renewed attention towards the mental health consequences of community life can be traced back to some seminal texts of sociology and reflects converging interests with other disciplines (including epidemiology, geography, and psychology). However, in reviewing research on place and health, Catalano and Pickett (2000: 64) observed that, even though scholars have written on this topic for over 150 years,

> contributors have rarely shown an awareness of the history and breadth of the work concerned with place and health. The result is that the field thrives for a period, stagnates, and begins again by duplicating much of what has gone before.

Regardless of whether one agrees with this assertion, the fact remains that few sources provide an overview of the long history and breadth of work on place (particularly neighborhoods and local places) and health. This is an area of research for which sociology and, in particular, mental health sociology has made important contributions.

The 20th anniversary of the American Sociological Association's Section on the Sociology of Mental Health provides an opportune time to reflect on this important history. Therefore, in the following pages, I will provide an overview of the

---

R.M. Carpiano (✉)
Department of Sociology, University of British Columbia, Vancouver, BC, Canada
e-mail: richard.carpiano@ubc.ca

past, current, and potential future contributions of sociology to understanding the mental health implications of local community life (namely, neighborhoods and other local residential areas or places). Motivated by the Shakespearean idea that "what is past is prologue," this chapter has two aims. The first aim is to provide the reader with an appreciation of research on local places and mental health. To achieve this, I map the genealogy of ideas in this research area—discussing research streams of sociological inquiry on local places and mental health over the past 20 years as well as seminal scholarship that dates back to the start of sociology as a formal discipline. In doing so, I intentionally avoid in-depth discussion of specific research findings as many extensive reviews already exist,[1] and limit my focus whenever possible to contributions from sociological research versus research in geography, epidemiology, psychology, community and social psychiatry, public health, and other disciplines.[2]

The second aim is to discuss future directions for research. For this, I build upon ideas reviewed in the historical overview in order to identify several key conceptual and substantive issues that are important for advancing sociology of mental health research on the consequences of local places.

5.1 Part 1: The Past as Prologue to the Present

The 1993 birth year of the Section on the Sociology of Mental Health provides a useful starting point for reviewing the longstanding history of research on the personal and collective health impacts of neighborhood and local residential environments—commonly termed "area (or neighborhood) health effects." As I will discuss below, a substantial amount of scholarship on place and health existed long before the 1990s. Nevertheless, I intentionally begin my historical review with 1993 because the Section's formation coincides with a period in health

---

[1] For readers looking for such reviews, there are many from which to choose—written by sociologists and scholars from other disciplines—that focus on health in general (e.g., Robert 1999), mental health (Hill and Maimon 2012), neighborhood effects research in general (Sampson et al. 2002) and life course issues regarding neighborhood health effects (Robert et al. 2010).

[2] To be sure, this is a tricky task given that (a) research on neighborhood health effects is a multi-disciplinary enterprise with other fields (most notably social epidemiology) commonly utilizing sociological concepts and theories and (b) sociologists publish this research in a variety of social science, public health, and psychiatry journals. Therefore, unlike a standard review article that aims to survey an entire area in breadth and depth, my historical overview and assessment of the field in terms of sociological emphases and contributions is heavily informed by scholarship published in the leading journals for medical sociologists, such as the *Journal of Health and Social Behavior* and *Social Science and Medicine*, as such forums are places for research that explicitly applies or informs sociological approaches to mental health. Furthermore, the high status of these forums is indicative of how scholars from sociology and other disciplines look to these sources for leading sociological ideas to inform their own work. Lastly, I intentionally exclude studies focused on rural-urban differences in mental health as well as the mental health effects of crowding, as such topics are outside the scope of this chapter.

research that witnessed the emergence of what can be considered the start of the current and, to date, most prolific period of this research focus. While many articles on place and health were published at this time, several seminal and highly cited articles authored or co-authored by sociologists deserve particular attention. In a 1993 article in the *Journal of Social Policy*, UK sociologist Sally Macintyre and her colleagues' argued for the need of health researchers to focus on people *and* places and study features of the local social and physical environment which might promote or inhibit health. Supporting their arguments were findings from their ongoing study of several, socioeconomically contrasting Scottish communities, which observed that variations in health across communities corresponded with—or mapped onto—between-area variation in local amenities, services, and hazards (see also MacIntyre and Ellaway 2000). Two years later, the journal *Health and Place* was founded, providing an interdisciplinary forum for this international research. By 1997, Robert Sampson et al. published in *Science* the results from their Chicago-wide community study of neighborhood collective efficacy and violent crime. Though focused more on a cause of poor mental and physical health than on an actual health outcome per se, this study's tremendous influence on health research can be attributed in major part to its application of multilevel regression models for estimating the effects of area- (ecologic) and individual-level processes on individual-level outcomes. The use of such multilevel analytic techniques (including the availability of software to apply them) would soon become commonplace in health research across multiple disciplines, including the sociology of mental health, thereby providing an important methodological tool for testing theoretically-driven hypotheses regarding meso-level (e.g., neighborhood) and macro-level (e.g., county, state/provincial, and national) structural conditions on personal health outcomes. But the contribution of Sampson et al.'s scholarship was not limited to their methodological approach. Their empirical findings regarding the mediating role of neighborhood collective efficacy—i.e. the extent to which residents in a neighborhood share similar values and are willing to take action for the collective good of others—for explaining the links between area social structural conditions (socioeconomic disadvantage and residential instability) and violent crime supported theoretical ideas on social disorganization developed decades earlier by the Chicago School of Sociology. As such, their theoretical and methodological approach would be subsequently applied by numerous health researchers—including mental health sociologists—to their own work in the years that followed.

By the time of Stephanie Robert's (1999) *Annual Review of Sociology* article on community socioeconomic context and health, the current era of research on neighborhood and local area health effects was well underway. At this time, however, sociological research on local places and mental health was relatively nascent compared to examinations of other health outcomes (e.g., physical conditions and mortality). Some mental health sociologists (e.g., Aneshensel and Sucoff 1996) and others (e.g., Driessen et al. 1998) had also started examining neighborhood context by this time. As evidenced by database search results, however, it would be a few more years before a critical mass of sociological scholarship would begin to emerge.

That such a lag in interest in neighborhoods and local places (hereafter, local places) existed in mental health sociology is curious given that, as I will detail below, some of the seminal studies in this area have focused on mental health.

5.1.1 From Classical Theory to the Chicago School

While the study of local place and mental health has evolved into a popular multi- and interdisciplinary research focus over the past 20 years, it is important to recognize that such current concerns only constitute the latest evolution of a research agenda that can be traced back to the early 20th century and the emergence of sociology as a formal discipline. In fact, the study of local place and mental health constitutes a critical link between the foundational scholarship of the discipline of sociology and longstanding research foci on social determinants of mental health— within the sociology of mental health as well as the interdisciplinary traditions of social and psychiatric epidemiology (see Bloom 2002). Hence, to put current research on local place and mental health in its proper historical context, it is necessary to go back several decades to the start of sociology as a formal discipline.

Discussion of the potential implications of social environments for mental well-being is not hard to find in the writings of some of the seminal scholars of Sociology—scholarship commonly read by most sociology graduate students. Perhaps the most cited example is Durkheim's (1951) use of observed geographic variation in suicide rates as empirical evidence for his theoretical suppositions regarding the consequences of social integration and regulation. Yet, Durkheim was not the only early sociologist who wrote of such links. Chronicling the unhealthy factory and living conditions faced by workers in the first half of the 1800s, Engels' ([1886] 2003) *Conditions of the Working Class in England*, recognizes the role of healthy environments for the mental well-being of children:

> it is unpardonable to sacrifice to the greed of an unfeeling bourgeoisie the time of children which should be devoted solely to their physical and mental development, and to withdraw them from school and the fresh air in order to wear them out for the benefit of the manufacturers. (p. 1246)

In his essay "The Metropolis and Mental Life," Simmel (1903 in Wolfe 1950) argued that inquiry into the meaning of modern social life must consider how environments or contexts such as the city structure the interplay between the personal self and the larger society in which the self is embedded. Specifically, Simmel compares urban and rural life and their implications for not simply differential lifestyles, but even personality—proposing that the "blasé attitude" or cognitive reserve common among city dwellers is an adaptation to (or psychological coping resource) for the numerous, pervasive stimuli of city environments that can bombard the senses.

Central to Simmel's arguments is an idea that pervaded much early sociological scholarship of the 19th and early 20th century (a historical period characterized by great societal transformations due to factors such as migration, technological development, secularization, and urbanization): cities, due to their geographic size, heterogeneity of people and cultures, and population density (among other factors), were fundamentally different from and, consequently, more pathological than rural places. As such, the urban environment was hypothesized to generate greater mental illness, crime, and deviant behavior than did rural localities. Such ideas by Simmel and others would influence the work of scholars affiliated with the Chicago "School" of Sociology in the first half of the twentieth century, who used Chicago as an urban laboratory for empirical sociological inquiry. The work of several Chicago scholars at this time (e.g., Robert Park and Ernest Burgess) identified variation across neighborhoods in terms of the prevalence of social phenomenon like social disorganization, crime and delinquency. Such investigations would inspire one of the most famous sociological studies of place and mental illness. In 1939, Robert Faris and H. Warren Dunham published *Mental Disorders in Urban Areas*, which applied Chicago School ideas to understanding the spatial distribution of mental illness. Their study tested hypotheses based on aspects of Burgess' Concentric Zone Theory, which aimed to understand the spatial patterning of social groups throughout urban areas. Analyzing data on patients admitted to psychiatric hospitals linked to their place of residence preadmission, the authors' found that rates of schizophrenia were higher in more central parts of Chicago (the poorer and most socially disorganized areas of the city) and decreased in magnitude as distance from the central city increased. By contrast, rates of bipolar disorder showed no similar pattern. Their ecological analysis limited inferences that could be made to individual cases and relied on hospital admission rates, not true prevalence. Yet, despite these limitations and the fact that other place and health studies had been conducted at the time of and long before this study (see Bloom 2002), Faris and Dunham's scholarship was influential in three ways. First and foremost, it stimulated a stream of multi-disciplinary mental health research focused specifically on the implications of neighborhood residential composition and other features of the local social environment (see March et al. 2008). Second, their conceptual focus on the relationship between social disorganization and mental illness would explicitly and implicitly underpin a significant amount of research on local place and mental health for subsequent decades through to the present day. Third, their work raised two key issues (or competing explanations) that would be centerpiece in studies of the social determinants of mental health up to the present day: social causation (that social conditions cause mental illness) and social selection or drift (that mental illness selects people into a particular social position) (Bloom 2002; March et al. 2008).

5.1.2 From Studying Places to Studying People

In addition to Faris and Dunham's influential findings (and replications of their findings by other authors, see e.g., Schroeder 1942) that warranted consideration of social environments as potential causes of mental illness, a body of empirical evidence was amassing that would have important implications for future research on the social determinants of mental health. Repeatedly, study findings were challenging the long-held assumption that urban places were more unhealthy (mentally or physically) than rural places and, as a result, researchers began to turn attention towards testing theories regarding how specific features or aspects of environments as well as personal social circumstances, such as socioeconomic status (SES), influenced mental health (Bloom 2002: 70–71). Two prominent examples of such foci included research co-authored by sociologists: The Midtown Manhattan Study, a community-based prevalence study of psychiatric illness initiated in 1952 that included sociologists Leo Srole and Thomas Langner among its primary members (Srole et al. 1962); and the New Haven (Connecticut) Study of social class and mental illness, which was conducted by sociologist August Hollingshead and psychiatrist Frederick Redlich (Hollingshead and Redlich 2007). Though both studies included geographic names in their respective titles, these were not studies of the role of place.

Also occurring at this time, however, was one noteworthy—though relatively less often discussed—prevalence study focused on how community and personal sociocultural environment contributed to mental disorder. The Stirling County Study investigated psychiatric disorder in a non-urban area of Nova Scotia that was selected as the study site due to the economic and cultural changes underway in the area. The study team of psychiatrists and social scientists was led by transcultural psychiatrist Alexander Leighton. Though most often viewed as one of many "true prevalence" studies of psychiatric epidemiology, the Stirling County Study's theoretical focus and multilevel, mixed-method design is particularly relevant for current day place and mental health research. With one of its central foci being the role of social disorganization as a contributing factor to mental illness rates, the Stirling County Study showed direct influences from Chicago School Sociology (Dohrenwend 1957; Hughes et al. 1960). In terms of methodology, the Study team conducted psychiatric interviews and reviewed medical records as well as developed and administered social survey instruments and undertook ethnographic observations. Noteworthy was the team's consideration of specific localities that were characterized by different ethnic and religious group composition (e.g., Francophone versus Anglophone communities) and degrees of social disorganization. Ultimately, the Stirling County Study found that rates of psychiatric disorder were higher overall in "disintegrated" (versus "integrated") communities—places categorized by the presence of "broken homes, few and weak associations, inadequate leadership, few recreational activities, hostility and inadequate communication, as well as poverty, secularization, and cultural confusion" (Leighton et al. 1963: 1021). Furthermore, lower class people living in integrated communities had less risk for disorder than upper class people in disintegrated communities (Leighton et al. 1963; Murphy 1994). Hence, the significance of the Stirling County Study for the study of place and health was its ability to take Faris and Dunham's work a step further by utilizing a design and analytic approach to test—and ultimately identify—significant socio-spatial variation in community (not hospitalization) rates of mental illness.

From the 1960s to the mid-1990s, multi- and interdisciplinary research on local place and mental health would appear in top psychiatric and social science journals (e.g., Leighton et al. 1971; Freeman 1978; Giggs 1986) and as book manuscripts [e.g., Scheper Hughes' (1979) ethnography of schizophrenia in rural Ireland]. However, compared to the current day, such publications were relatively sporadic.

This multi-decade lack of focus on neighborhoods and local communities by sociologists studying mental health was ironic for two reasons raised by Silver et al. (2002). First, by the 1960s, deinstitutionalization was underway and individuals with mental health problems were now residing and being treated in the community rather than in institutions. Hence, a concerted focus by sociologists on local place and mental would have been fruitful for both academic and applied purposes. Second, this time period saw the rise of scholarship on social stress and mental health, which is a core area in mental health sociology that persists to the current day—the origins of which could be traced back to Faris and Dunham's work but was a key focus in later seminal research such as the Midtown Manhattan Study. Rather than focusing on environments directly, social stress researchers focused on personal socioeconomic status (SES) as a key indicator of one's social context, including residential social environment (even though personal SES is an inadequate indicator of neighborhood SES). Such a de-emphasis on environments was unfortunate. Incidentally, Leighton et al. (1963), in discussing their Stirling County findings (summarized above), make a final recommendation that highlights the importance of both considering person and place:

> It is not poverty or limited education or lower class status, per se, that makes the difference to mental health, but rather a whole group of factors that tend to be associated with these and that create a social environment that lacks features that are vitally important to mental health. To improve mental health, economic resources must be mobilized up to a point, education must be provided up to a point, but this will not be enough unless these factors bring with them the other environmental forces which add up to giving the individual the feeling that he is a worthwhile member of a worthwhile group (p. 1026).

A broad database search for relevant publications during this time period revealed few related studies on place and mental health published in either *Social Science and Medicine* or the *Journal of Health and Social Behavior* (*JHSB*, and its original title, *Journal of Health and Human Behavior*)—long two major forums for publishing key research foci within mental health and medical sociology. In fact, one study on neighborhood context and mental health published in *JHSB* by Kasl and Harburg (1975) was fairly dismissive of ecological studies of mental health in the tradition of Faris and Dunham, arguing that:

> A scanning of the relevant literature on mental health and the urban environment reveals a surprisingly small amount of evidence that is fairly interpretable and can be evaluated regarding the possible impact of neighborhood and residential parameters on mental health and well-being. (p. 278)

Analyzing data from a sample of respondents residing in four Detroit census tracts, Kasl and Harburg interpreted their own findings regarding census tract characteristics, respondents' personal perceptions of the neighborhood, and mental health outcomes as raising further doubt about the role of local residential context for mental health—concluding that the findings of the many prior ecologic studies "have not really implicated the urban environment in any convincing way" (p. 280). While it can certainly be argued (particularly with the benefit of nearly 40 years of theoretical and methodological advancements) that Kasl and Harburg's (1975) findings and analytic approach raise more doubts than conclusive answers about the etiological nature of neighborhood contexts, their concern with ecologic studies of mental illness was certainly valid. The concern for committing an ecologic fallacy—the risk of drawing inaccurate conclusions about individuals from results based on data measured at higher (ecologic) levels of analysis or aggregation such as at the neighborhood level (Robinson 1950)—would continue to plague studies of place and health until the 1990s. Ecological approaches have long been regarded as inferior to individual level studies (Schwartz 1994, see also Macintye and Ellaway 2000). Related to this belief was the thinking that ecologic variables do not cause disease (Schwartz 1994). Only recently has such logic come to be challenged.

5.1.3 The Current Era of Neighborhood Mental Health Effects

By the 1990s, conceptual and methodological thinking about ecologic processes would reinvigorate study of place and health. Conceptually, there were calls in a variety of health disciplines (e.g., epidemiology, geography, medical sociology, and health psychology) to reconsider the role of ecologic factors. MacIntyre and Ellaway (2000) attribute this paradigmatic turnabout to several coinciding factors in related disciplines. Within epidemiology, there emerged critiques regarding the individualistic focus in chronic disease epidemiology and calls for refocusing attention on populations and ecologic influences (e.g., Schwartz 1994). Within medical geography, a call was made for re-emphasizing "place" (e.g., see Kearns and Joseph 1993; Curtis and Rees Jones 1998). Within sociology, there was recognition of the limits of an individualistically-oriented epidemiological paradigm in the study of health inequalities (MacIntyre and Ellaway 2000; see also Robert 1999) as well as the influence of work in urban sociology focused on neighborhood inequality that would be cited extensively by medical sociologists (e.g., Wilson 1987). In sum, there was appreciation that while these and other health disciplines acknowledged the role of "upstream" (contextual) causes of health, most studies considered their role only through individual life circumstances (e.g., SES, race/ethnicity) (MacIntyre and Ellaway 2000: 337).

Methodologically, the development and accessibility of multilevel modeling (MLM) approaches and software greatly enabled this reconsideration of ecologic factors in empirical research. Researchers could now more easily test hypotheses regarding the relationship between neighborhood-level conditions like poverty and social disorganization and individual-level mental health while controlling for individual-level confounding factors. While such tests could be conducted previously under certain sampling conditions via the use of traditional regression techniques, MLM approaches offered the ability to examine between- and within-neighborhood variance in mental health outcomes among respondents clustered by neighborhood location.

As noted earlier, mental health sociology entered this emerging wave of neighborhood effects research a bit later than other health areas; however, the resulting contributions, as discussed below, have been quite prolific and insightful. Overall, this scholarship has shown obvious ties to the work of Faris and Dunham as well as the Chicago School of Sociology. Some of the earliest studies identified that neighborhood-level socioeconomic disadvantage and residential stability had independent associations with individual-level mental health (e.g., depressive symptoms, major depressive disorder, and substance abuse disorder) net of the effects of individual-level characteristics (e.g., Ross 2000; Silver et al. 2002), thereby addressing a major criticism of Faris and Dunham's pioneering ecologic analysis.

While neighborhood health effects research has been a multi- and interdisciplinary enterprise, a major contribution of the sociology of mental health—that is, scholarship that applies an explicitly sociological theoretical approach to studying mental health—to this enterprise has been the investigation of a variety of theoretically-motivated mediating and moderating pathways through which neighborhood context may influence personal mental health. A now substantial corpus of existing (and quite exciting) work has examined pathways such as stress (e.g., Aneshensel and Sucoff 1996), health behaviors (e.g., Hale et al. 2013), and access to coping resources (including how neighborhoods may enhance or undermine the resources people have to maintain mental well-being in daily life (e.g., Christie-Mazell and Erickson 2007; Carpiano and Kimbro 2012). Below, I highlight three particular research streams that have emerged in mental health sociology research. Each of these streams has raised important ideas for furthering research on neighborhood health effects on mental as well as physical health outcomes—ideas that bridge ideas from each of the streams. Hence, for all three areas, I also discuss how this scholarship has existing or potential linkages with related research on physical health and other health-related outcomes.

5.1.4 Neighborhood Stressors

The stress process model has long been a major focus of the sociology of mental health (particularly for understanding how personal SES impacts mental health). In recent years, this model has commonly been utilized as a way to theorize linkages between person and place—thereby situating micro-level experiences of an individual within the meso-level social context of neighborhood (e.g., Pearlin 1999; Aneshensel 2010). In particular, a significant amount of research using this stress approach has focused on perceptions that an individual has of the social and physical disorder in the neighborhood, such as the perceived presence of features such as crime, lack of safety, incivility or lack of cohesion among neighbors, graffiti/ vandalism, and abandoned buildings. These cues may be perceived by individuals as signs of a breakdown of social order and control in the neighborhood and thus result in a stressful and threatening environment that undermines mental health (e.g., Geis and Ross 1998; Christie-Mizell and Erickson 2007; Ross 2011). To date, a number of studies have found evidence that such subjective factors mediate some or all of the observed association between specific neighborhood objective conditions (i.e. measured using neighborhood-level census data) and mental health outcomes among adults (Ross 2000) and adolescents (Aneshensel and Sucoff 1996). Further work examining specific responses to such features has found that perceived disorder is associated with increased features of alienation (increased powerlessness, isolation, and mistrust), which, in turn, leads to increased anxiety, anger, and depression (e.g., Geis and Ross 1998; Ross and Mirowsky 2009). Additionally, the connection between neighborhood disadvantage and anger has also been found to be contingent upon social comparisons—specifically, how residents believe their income compares to that of their neighbors (Schieman et al. 2006). Collectively, this work argues that the link between objective conditions and personal distress is mediated by one's cognitions (the subjective interpretations of the environment) and emotions (subjective alienation and anger) (Ross 2011).

Nevertheless, recent scholarship challenges some of the abovementioned emphasis on perceptions or cognitions as a key mechanism linking neighborhood social disorder and mental health. Specifically, Turner et al.'s (2013) examination of the mental health of youth ages 10–17 indicates that exposure to *actual* (i.e. experienced) violence and victimization as well as family social support have a more substantial role in explaining the link between social disorder and mental health than has been previously assumed.

Further informing this emerging debate about perceived and actual neighborhood experiences and conditions are Turney et al.'s (2013) insightful qualitative findings from the Moving to Opportunity (MTO) randomized housing experiment for relocating low income families from high to low poverty neighborhoods. Consistent with research focused on cognitions, adults in the experimental condition of moving to low poverty neighborhoods reported experiencing increased personal self-worth, mastery, and motivation for improvement that they attributed to observing and emulating their (mostly homeowner) neighbors—people whom respondents often and with pride described as "respectable," "decent," and "hardworking" (Turney et al. 2013: 11). Yet, consistent with research on experiencing actual conditions, experimentals also reported increased stress from features such as violence-related victimization (e.g., in cases whether neighborhood conditions declined over time) and inadequate services (e.g., public transportation), but reduced parenting stress and worry due to the presence of other adults looking out for the safety and welfare of the local children. Hence, these collective results show the need to consider a holistic view of how neighborhoods produce stress via multiple mechanisms.

All things considered, when taking a broad view of this stress-focused approach—i.e. one that transcends debates about whether specific explanations or mechanisms are complementary or competing—the ideas generated from this scholarship have great complementarity with research that investigates how objective and perceived neighborhood social conditions influence personal stress biomarkers (e.g., cortisol) (e.g., Karb et al. 2012) and other health-related outcomes. For example, several studies have identified a substantial effect of recent exposure to neighborhood homicides on the cognitive test score performance of African American children (Sharkey 2010) as well as the attention, impulse control, and vocabulary assessments of preschool children (Sharkey et al. 2012). For this latter study, some evidence suggests parental psychological distress as a mediating factor between homicide exposure and child outcomes—findings that align with Turner et al.'s (2013) abovementioned results regarding family social support as a disorder-mental health mediator. Hence, the abovementioned neighborhood stressor studies provide insights that extend well beyond mental health to broader knowledge of health and general well-being.

5.1.5 The Interplay of Neighborhoods with Other Social Contexts

While much of the stress-focused research has examined the ways in which neighborhoods as meso-level contexts generate stress that undermines coping resources and mental health, recent studies have also sought to conceptualize neighborhoods not simply as environments that people inhabit and that subsequently expose them to mental health risks via social disorder or other local stressors, but as one particular social context that has overlap with other social contexts in which people are situated—all of which have mental health implications. Whereas the abovementioned neighborhood stress research has been heavily influenced by the stress process model, this work draws more heavily on community sociology approaches to understanding how neighborhoods matter—particularly social capital and social disorganization theoretical traditions. This latter perspective, which has its roots in the Chicago School, considers how neighborhood structural characteristics, such as socioeconomic disadvantage and residential instability, affect collective and personal outcomes via undermining community social organization—i.e. the extent of informal and formal networks and their ability to realize common goals and maintain effective controls (Sampson and Groves 1989). These elements of social organization are often referred to in the health literature as features of collective efficacy and social capital (see Carpiano 2006). To date, such approaches have examined a range of mental health-related outcomes.

For example, in terms of adolescent mental health, Maimon et al. (2010) applied ideas from Durkheim and social disorganization theory to examine the interplay of neighborhood and family for preventing adolescent suicide. Their findings revealed that neighborhood collective efficacy (neighborhood social cohesion and informal social control) enhanced the protective effect of family attachment for adolescent suicide risk.

Focusing on adult mental health, Haines et al. (2011) combined ideas from two foci of mental health sociology research (and two conceptions of community): neighborhoods and general social networks. They found that the relationship between neighborhood disadvantage and depressive symptoms was mediated by general network social capital even after controlling for perceived neighborhood disorder examined commonly in other studies.

Finally, in terms of resources for coping with parenting stressors, Carpiano and Kimbro (2012) tested ideas from community and family sociology regarding the role of neighborhood social capital as a resource for female caregivers of children. Their results indicated that neighborhood social capital moderated the negative association between parenting strain and mastery and that this buffering effect was further contingent upon the degree to which one socialized with neighbors and thus had access to such neighborhood resources. Similar findings were reported by Turney et al. (2013) in their qualitative study of MTO participants' mental health.

Collectively, these and similar studies focusing on a variety of health outcomes (e.g., Carpiano et al. 2011; Moore et al. 2011; Kelly et al. 2012; Verhaeghe and Tampubolon 2012) highlight the utility of considering the interplay of neighborhood context with other social contexts in which people are embedded in their daily lives (e.g., family/household, friendship networks, jobs, and other social domains). Such an approach considers the modern day role and relative importance of neighborhoods for different types of people and the social circumstances they face in their daily lives.

5.1.6 Lifecourse Processes

A third area considers lifecourse processes—specifically, the interaction of people and places over time. While the majority of neighborhood health effects research measures both neighborhood context and personal outcomes at one point in time, research has now begun to examine the effects of neighborhood context over time (i.e. at specific stages of one's lifecourse). In one of the first studies to investigate this issue, Wheaton and Clark (2003) proposed and tested a conceptual model that considered the role of neighborhood disadvantage during childhood and early adulthood in the generation of stressors as well as childhood, adolescent, and early adult mental health outcomes (internalizing and externalizing problems). Their results indicated that current neighborhood disadvantage had no effect on early adult mental health. Rather, the earlier (childhood) neighborhood context had both lagged and cumulative effects on current mental health. Furthermore, the mental health effect of neighborhood context was contingent on the extent of family SES, highlighting an important issue for broader research on SES and mental health: "The proper specification of the individual-level social class effect on mental health requires consideration of the interdependence between individual and contextual components of social class" (p. 702).

Though research examining neighborhood context at multiple time points is still more the exception than the norm, further work is underway. In particular, two recent studies focused on child development outcomes reported lagged effects of childhood neighborhood disadvantage on later verbal ability (Sampson et al. 2008) and reading comprehension outcomes (Lloyd et al. 2010). Another study has identified multigenerational effects of neighborhood poverty on child cognitive ability (Sharkey and Elwert 2011). These findings all have implications for selecting children into low SES in adulthood, which, in turn, can result in greater risk for subsequent mental health outcomes. Complementing this work is Vartanian and Houser's (2010) sibling fixed effects analysis of 38 years of longitudinal data, which found that growing up in an advantaged neighborhoods had long term health effects, but neighborhood context in adulthood had little to no health effect. Collectively, this work highlights the importance of considering how neighborhood context matters at specific "critical periods" of development and cumulatively over the lifecourse (see Robert et al. 2010 for a thorough treatment of this topic) as well as the inter-relationship of neighborhood-level and individual-level selection and causation processes over the lifecourse.

5.2 Part 2: The Present as Prologue to the Future

As indicated by the studies discussed above, a major contribution of mental health sociology—and sociology in general—to this multi- and inter-disciplinary field of research has been the application of thoughtful theoretical considerations regarding how neighborhood environments "matter" for mental health. In essence, such application is consistent with Link's (2008) call for an "epidemiological sociology" approach to studying the role of social factors for disease etiology that applies knowledge from the diverse range of subareas within sociology. Indeed, the study of local place and mental health has witnessed many sociological ideas being adopted and utilized by researchers in other disciplines such as social epidemiology. In light of this approach, I offer several recommendations for furthering future research—all of which have important implications for building and testing theories about local places and mental health.

5.2.1 Conceptualizing Theoretical Mechanisms: For Whom and for What?

Going forward, it is important for the sociology of mental health to remain cognizant in its theorizing about two issues regarding how local places might matter: (1) For whom? and (2) For what?

By "For whom?" I refer to the need to consider carefully the specific population that is to be examined. To date, this research has most commonly examined the role of specific factors on a general population, such as adults or adolescents. As a result, the findings (or in the case of quantitative studies, the slope estimate for a particular variable) is the average effect of a neighborhood condition (e.g., poverty, collective efficacy) on an outcome. While such average effects are important from a population health standpoint, they can mask important subgroup variation. Hence, focusing on specific demographic groups offers useful intellectual and practical insights. Different demographic groups have different uses for and exposures to neighborhood environments as well as different rates of specific mental health problems. For example, in addition to children and adolescents, certain adults may be more likely to spend greater time in a neighborhood than others (e.g., people who work full-time) and thus have greater exposure to the health promoting and health damaging aspects of the local environment. Such groups include, but are not limited to female caregivers of children (given that women are more often the primary caregiver of a child and more likely to be a stay-at-home parent than men), the elderly, and the unemployed—three groups that each face unique mental health risks due to their social positions based on gender, age, and SES. Hence, testing a specific theoretically-driven mechanism on one or more subpopulations for which such a mechanism may factor prominently (or, in the case of comparison groups, differentially) can improve understanding of the many unique ways that specific neighborhood contextual features might undermine or promote mental health (e.g., see Christie-Mizell and Erickson 2007; Aneshensel et al. 2011). After all, while specific conditions may matter in certain ways for mental health, it is unlikely that they may matter in similar ways for all residents.

By "For what?" I refer to carefully considering the outcome to be examined in light of the neighborhood process of interest. If it can be conjectured that a certain neighborhood process matters for health (mental and/or physical health), then for what outcome(s) should we see its positive or negative effects manifest (and through which pathways)? This issue has been raised previously with respect to the stress model (Thoits 1995), but has validity regardless of the theoretical framework used. For example, might we expect some neighborhood conditions to have greater implications for psychological distress versus clinical levels of depression or for internalizing versus externalizing problems? Likewise, what neighborhood conditions might be "double-edged swords" for mental health—i.e. useful for preventing the onset of certain conditions, but presenting risk for others? Such considerations require researchers to maintain a healthy skepticism of community life—i.e. viewing it as a social phenomenon and not automatically as a potential panacea for personal and collective ills (e.g., see Carpiano 2008).

Central to answering these two questions and to a priori theorizing overall is the need to carefully reflect on potential intervening neighborhood- and individual-level mechanisms linking an outcome to the local environment, such as local amenities, stressors, personal health behaviors, and even conditions in the home (marital quality, parenting) and beyond the neighborhood itself (work, family, networks). In an effort to facilitate these considerations in building theories, I offer below some substantive ideas from other areas of sociology that can be beneficial for constructing empirically testable mechanistic explanations and advancing this area of research.

5.2.2 Thinking Organizationally

To date, sociological research on neighborhood mental health effects has overwhelmingly focused on two aspects of objective (versus perceived) neighborhood social conditions: social structural conditions in general (e.g., neighborhood SES and residential stability) and features of neighborhood social organization (i.e. the extent and quality of interactions among neighbors and the resources or social capital that inhere in such ties). Such foci explicitly center attention on the people living in a neighborhood and the concentration (and potential sharing) of economic, cultural, and social capital. But it is important to recognize that neighborhoods consist of more than just the people who live there. Neighborhoods are also locations for organizations that have potentially important implications for promoting local quality of life, preventing the development of mental health problems and helping those with mental health problems via treatment and other (non-health-related) services (McQuarrie and Marwell 2009; Metraux et al. 2007).

Sociologists studying local place and mental health have drawn many theoretical and empirical ideas from community and urban sociology—yet surprisingly, have paid very little attention to neighborhood-based organizations, such as community centers, non-profit organizations, child care centers, and social service agencies, among many others that provide formal services and programs for local residents. Within recent years, community and urban sociology has developed a keen interest in understanding how neighborhood and other local organizations serve as sources of instrumental and other resources for communities, individuals, and families (see Allard and Small 2013). Some notable examples include Small's (2009) study of the role of child care centers for assisting families as well as facilitating the building of social capital among parents and Dominguez and Watkins' (2003) study of single mothers, which identified the important roles of social service organizations for linking these women to social support as well as job assistance programs.

Such considerations of local organizations and services can be quite informative for many key issues in the sociology of mental health. From the basic standpoint of social support, research on the sociology of mental health—particularly research applying the stress paradigm—has focused heavily on the role of support from informal ties (family, friends, and neighbors). Nevertheless, it is important from academic and practice/policy perspectives to recognize that many formal services exist to provide resources that might otherwise be unavailable to people who need them. This situation is particularly relevant for socially disadvantaged communities, where social capital among neighbors may be weak or less valuable for addressing specific personal and collective needs. As such, more focused attention on the roles of such organizations—many of which are often located near to the populations they aim to serve—can not only provide greater insight into the role of local community life for mental health, but provide an improved disciplinary link between community and urban sociology and the sociology of mental health. Furthermore, it can help to facilitate an improved interaction between mental health sociology and mental health geography, which has had a longstanding focus on the socio-spatial distribution of mental health treatment and related services and the development of "service dependent ghettos" (see the extensive review by Wolch and Philo 2000)

5.2.3 The Role of Neighborhood Culture

The role of culture in the study of local place and mental health dates back to Faris and Dunham (1939) and is featured prominently in later work by others (e.g., Leighton et al. 1963; Scheper-Hughes 1979) who specifically looked at culture as something that was contextual (i.e. part of the environment). More recently, however, few examples exist of sociological investigations of neighborhood culture and mental health aside from examinations of neighborhood social cohesion and informal social control (often combined into a single measure of collective efficacy). Even health research on ethnic and other neighborhood enclaves, which often focuses on culture as a major factor, often does not directly measure culture—in large part due to limitations of existing data sources.

Culture has importance both for thinking about causes of poor mental health (e.g., local racism or heterosexism) and the generation of resources to cope with such causes (e.g., attitudes towards healthy and unhealthy health risk behaviors, collective efficacy). It also matters for residents' appraisals and meanings of specific situations, which, to date have been examined from an individualistic, social psychological standpoint common within stress research. While not all stressors are neighborhood-specific (something often not explicitly considered in neighborhood mental health effects research), the study of culture within neighborhoods and local communities provides a way to contextualize the appraisals of and responses to a variety of intra- and extra-neighborhood phenomenon and experiences not simply limited to stressors, such as immigrant acculturation (a popular focal area in health research) (Kimbro 2009).

In light of these issues, mental health sociology can benefit from community and urban sociologists' renewed interest in the role of culture. This work has utilized a number of useful conceptual tools for conducting rigorous empirical analyses of how cultural processes contribute to personal and collective action [see Lamont and Small's (2008) review of the ways in which culture has been examined in the study of poverty (an area that often considers neighborhood context)]. In an interesting quantitative application to studying the consequences of neighborhood disadvantage for adolescents, Harding (2007) found greater heterogeneity of cultural frames (schema for interpreting the world) and scripts for action in disadvantaged versus advantaged neighborhoods and that, in such heterogeneous (or culturally diverse) places, adolescents were less likely to act in ways that were consistent with their own frames and scripts (with respect to romantic relationships and the consequences of teenage pregnancy). Such ideas and findings lead to no shortage of possibilities for studying the role of local places for mental health—including but certainly not limited to the studying the collective (versus personal) interpretation/appraisal of local stressors, identifying specific symptoms, choosing among different coping responses (essentially cultural scripts), and, from the perspective of modified labeling theory and stigma research (Link and Phelan 2001), managing daily life with a particular mental health condition. Furthermore, such approaches offer great utility for furthering study on racial/ethnic differences in mental health, considering that race/ethnicity is often used as a crude measure of culture despite significant within-group cultural heterogeneity (Lamont and Small 2008).

5.2.4 Health Behaviors: Neighborhood Structure and Personal Agency

Though numerous studies have examined how neighborhood conditions are associated with personal health behaviors, such as smoking, binge drinking, drug use, and sexual behavior (e.g., Kimbro 2009; Carpiano 2008; Carpiano et al. 2011; Kelly et al. 2012), few studies have specifically examined health behaviors as mediators and moderators between the local conditions and mental health outcomes (see Hill and Maimon 2012).

Given calls for better understanding the role of personal agency in neighborhood health effects research (Robert et al. 2010), future examinations of health behaviors as risk factors and coping mechanisms for mental health problems would be well served by incorporating ideas from recent scholarship on health lifestyles (Frohlich et al. 2002; Cockerham 2005). This emerging area of research, which draws from the sociological theories of Max Weber on lifestyles and Pierre Bourdieu on capitals and habitus, aims to better understand how such seemingly individualistic, discrete behaviors (as they have long been treated in health research) can be better understood when conceptualized and empirically investigated as social practices that emanate from the relationship between personal agency and social structure. For example, in their mixed methods study of youth smoking, Frohlich et al. (2002) found that, though smoking-discouraging resources were more prevalent in high versus low SES communities, the social practices of youth with regard to smoking were not always consistent with the social structural features of these communities—thereby indicating variation in how people interact with the social structure and implicating the need to consider the interplay between structure and agency for understanding health outcomes. Such considerations offer the opportunity to not only better understand the links between neighborhood context, health behaviors, and mental health, but to also improve overall how we theorize and empirically study specific neighborhood-based mechanisms.

5.2.5 Neighborhoods as Settings for Labeling, Stigma, and the Lived Experience of Mental Illness

The vast majority of sociological scholarship on local place and mental health applies a social causation approach: how local conditions can generate mental illness among residents. Though substantial attention is given in this research to "ruling out" selection effects or explanations (people with mental illnesses moving into disadvantaged neighborhoods), it is surprising that sociological research rarely considers and examines the implications of local places for people who already have a mental illness [for two exceptions, see Segal et al. (1980) examination of neighborhood types and community reaction to persons with mental illnesses and Metraux et al.'s (2007) study of residential segregation in Philadelphia among Medicaid recipients with psychiatric disability]. Research on the lived experiences of mental illness, including scholarship on labeling and stigma (Link and Phelan 2001), strongly implicates the everyday social experiences of people with mental health problems—particularly their interactions with others who may, upon knowing of one's condition, avoid or even discriminate against them. Consequently, future research on the consequences of labeling and stigma should consider the local places that persons with mental illness occupy in their daily routines, as such locations may certainly have implications for understanding the course of a condition, prospects for successfully coping with the condition, and overall quality of life while living with the condition. Essentially, such work necessitates considering the relationship between selection and causation processes—asking the question: while people with mental illness may select into specific neighborhoods, how do the conditions of these neighborhoods matter for these people's long term outcomes in terms of experiences of discrimination and resource access?

5.3 Conclusion

This chapter has aimed to provide an introductory primer and appreciation of sociological contributions to the study of local place and mental health. My goal was to not only highlight intellectual foundations of and recent contributions to this area of inquiry, but to identify potential future advances that could arise from constructing and testing mechanistic explanations informed by ideas from other areas of health- and non-health-related inquiry. Such a task helps critically examine Catalano and Pickett's (2000: 64) assertion that, within the broad area of study on place and health, authors have rarely shown an awareness of the history and breadth of scholarship on this topic and, as a result, the field thrives, stagnates, and resurges—"duplicating much of what has gone before." In reviewing the historical evolution of sociological research on local place and mental health and its interplay with other related areas of sociomedical inquiry, some conclusions can be made about why there was stagnation and now an impressive resurgence of interest in this topic. Furthermore, the recent development of different streams of research within this area certainly show close ties to longstanding approaches in mental health sociology and sociology overall—as well as great potential for establishing new ties to other exciting research areas. However, rather than simply rehashing old concepts, these recent developments represent modern-day applications and further refinements of prior scholarship that, in turn, have furthered this decades-old research focus and broadened—not duplicated—our understanding of the many ways in which local places matters for mental health (and health in general). All areas of scholarship enjoy periods of thriving and stagnation. Regardless of how long this field's current enthusiasm will be sustained or stay "en vogue," a continued epidemiological sociology approach to studying the etiology of mental illness—that is, an approach that utilizes a wide breadth of ideas from different areas of sociology—will ensure the continued influx of fresh ideas for building, testing, and refining theory, resulting in novel contributions to this multi-disciplinary area of study as well as research on social determinants of mental health overall.

Acknowledgments I authored this work while receiving funding from Investigator Awards from the Michael Smith Foundation for Health Research and the Canadian Institutes of Health Research. I express sincere thanks to Stephanie Robert and Margaret Weden, who through many fruitful e-mail exchanges on this topic facilitated some of my thinking in preparing several parts of this chapter (whether they realize it or not). All the assertions and conclusions as well as any errors and omissions in this chapter, however, are solely my own.

References

Allard, S. W., & Small, M. L. (2013). Reconsidering the urban disadvantaged: The role of systems, institutions, and organizations. *The Annals of the American Academy of Political and Social Science, 647*, 6–20.

Aneshensel, C. S. (2010). Neighborhood as a social context of the stress process. In W. R. Avison, C. S. Aneshensel, S. Schieman, & B. Wheaton (Eds.), *Advances in the stress process: Essays in honor of Leonard I. Pearlin* (pp. 35–52). New York: Springer.

Aneshensel, C. S., Ko, M. J., Chodosh, J., & Wight, R. G. (2011). The urban neighborhood and cognitive functioning in late middle age. *Journal of Health and Social Behavior, 52*(2), 163–179.

Aneshensel, C. S., & Sucoff, C. (1996). The neighborhood context of adolescent mental health. *Journal of Health and Social Behavior, 37*, 293–310.

Bloom, S. W. (2002). *The word as scalpel: A history of medical sociology*. New York: Oxford University Press.

Carpiano, R. M. (2006). Towards a neighborhood-based resource theory of social capital for health: Can bourdieu and sociology help? *Social Science and Medicine, 62*(1), 165–175.

Carpiano, R. M. (2008). Actual or potential neighborhood resources and access to them: Testing hypotheses of social capital for the health of female caregivers. *Social Science and Medicine, 67*(4), 568–582.

Carpiano, R. M., Kelly, B. C., Easterbrook, A., & Parsons, J. T. (2011). Community and drug use among gay men the role of neighborhoods and networks. *Journal of Health and Social Behavior, 52*(1), 74–90.

Carpiano, R. M., & Kimbro, R. T. (2012). Neighborhood social capital, parenting strain, and personal mastery among female primary caregivers of children. *Journal of Health and Social Behavior, 53*(2), 232–247.
Catalano, R., & Pickett, K. E. (2000). A taxonomy of research concerned with place and health. In G. L. Albrecht, R. Fitzpatrick, & S. C. Scrimshaw (Eds.), *Handbook of social studies in health and medicine* (pp. 64–84). Thousand Oaks, California: Sage.
Christie-Mizell, C. A., & Erickson, R. J. (2007). Mothers and mastery: The consequences of perceived neighborhood disorder. *Social Psychology Quarterly, 70*(4), 340–365.
Cockerham, W. C. (2005). Health lifestyle theory and the convergence of agency and structure. *Journal of Health and Social Behavior, 46*(1), 51–67.
Curtis, S., & Rees Jones, I. (1998). Is there a place for geography in the analysis of health inequality? *Sociology of Health & Illness, 20*(5), 645–672.
Dohrenwend, B. P. (1957). The Stirling County Study: A research program on relations between sociocultural factors and mental illness. *American Psychologist, 12*(2), 78–85.
Dominguez, S., & Watkins, C. (2003). Creating networks for survival and mobility: Social capital among African-American and Latin-American low-income mothers. *Social Problems, 50*(1), 111–135.
Driessen, G., Gunther, N., & Van Os, J. (1998). Shared social environment and psychiatric disorder: A multilevel analysis of individual and ecological effects. *Social Psychiatry and Psychiatric Epidemiology, 33*(12), 606–612.
Durkheim, E. (1951). *Suicide*. New York: The Free Press.
Engels, F. (2003). The condition of the working class in England. *American Journal of Public Health, 93*(8), 1246–1249.
Faris, R. E. L., & Dunham, H. W. (1939). *Mental disorders in urban areas: An ecological study of schizophrenia and other psychoses*. Chicago, Illinois: University of Chicago Press.
Freeman, H. (1978). Mental health and the environment. *British Journal of Psychiatry, 132*, 113–124.
Frohlich, K. L., Potvin, L., Chabot, P., & Corin, E. (2002). A theoretical and empirical analysis of context: Neighbourhoods, smoking and youth. *Social Science and Medicine, 54*(9), 1401–1417.
Geis, K. J., & Ross, C. E. (1998). A new look at urban alienation: The effect of neighborhood disorder on perceived powerlessness. *Social Psychology Quarterly, 61*, 232–246.
Giggs, J. A. (1986). Mental disorders and ecological structure in Nottingham. *Social Science and Medicine, 23*(10), 945–961.
Haines, V. A., Beggs, J. J., & Hurlbert, J. S. (2011). Neighborhood disadvantage, network social capital, and depressive symptoms. *Journal of Health and Social Behavior, 52*(1), 58–73.
Hale, L., Hill, T. D., Elliot Friedman, F., Nieto, J., Galvao, L. W., Engelman, C., et al. (2013). Perceived neighborhood quality, sleep quality, and health status: Evidence from the survey of the health of wisconsin. *Social Science and Medicine, 79*, 16–22.
Harding, D. J. (2007). Cultural context, sexual behavior, and romantic relationships in disadvantaged neighborhoods. *American Sociological Review, 72*(3), 341–364.
Hill, T., & Maimon, D. (2012). Neighborhood context and mental health. In C. S. Aneshensel, J. C. Phelan, & A. Bierman (Eds.), *Handbook of the sociology of mental health* (2nd ed., pp. 479–501). New York: Springer.
Hollingshead, A., & Redlich, F. (2007). Social class and mental illness: A community study. *American Journal of Public Health*.
Hughes, C. C., Tremblay, M. A., Rapoport, R. N., & Leighton, A. H. (1960). *People of cove and woodlot: Communities from the standpoint of social psychiatry, volume II: The Stirling County Study of psychiatric disorder and sociocultural environment*. New York: Basic Books.
Karb, R. A., Elliott, M. R., Dowd, J. B., & Morenoff, J. D. (2012). Neighborhood-level stressors, social support, and diurnal patterns of cortisol: The Chicago Community adult health study. *Social Science and Medicine, 75*(6), 1038–1047.

Kasl, S. V., & Harburg, E. (1975). Mental health and the urban environment: Some doubts and second thoughts. *Journal of Health and Social Behavior, 16*(3), 268–282.

Kearns, R. A., & Joseph, A. E. (1993). Space in its place: Developing the link in medical geography. *Social Science and Medicine, 37*(6), 711–717.

Kelly, B. C., Carpiano, R. M., Easterbrook, A., & Parsons, J. T. (2012). Sex and the community: The implications of neighbourhoods and social networks for sexual risk behaviours among urban gay men. *Sociology of Health and Illness, 34*(7), 1085–1102.

Kimbro, R. T. (2009). Acculturation in context: Gender, age at migration, neighborhood ethnicity, and health behaviors. *Social Science Quarterly, 90*(5), 1145–1166.

Lamont, M., & Small, M. L. (2008). How culture matters: Enriching our understanding of poverty. In D. Harris & A. Lin (Eds.), *The colors of poverty: Why racial and ethnic disparities persist* (pp. 76–102). New York: Russell Sage.

Leighton, D. C., Hagnell, O., Leighton, A. H., Harding, J. S., Kellert, S. R., & Danley, R. A. (1971). Psychiatric disorder in a Swedish and a Canadian community: An exploratory study. *Social Science and Medicine, 5*(3), 189–209.

Leighton, D. C., Harding, J. S., Macklin, D. B., Hughes, C. C., & Leighton, A. H. (1963). Psychiatric findings of the Stirling County Study. *American Journal of Psychiatry, 119*, 1021–1026.

Link, B. G. (2008). Epidemiological sociology and the social shaping of population health. *Journal of Health and Social Behavior, 49*(4), 367–384.

Link, B. G., & Phelan, J. C. (2001). Conceptualizing stigma. *Annual Review of Sociology, 27*, 363–385.

Lloyd, J. E. V., Li, L., & Hertzman, C. (2010). Early experiences matter: Lasting effect of concentrated disadvantage on children's language and cognitive outcomes. *Health and Place, 16*(2), 371–380.

MacIntyre, S., & Ellaway, A. (2000). Ecological approaches: Rediscovering the role of the physical and social environment. In L. F. Berkman & I. Kawachi (Eds.), *Social Epidemiology* (pp. 332–348). New York: Oxford University Press.

MacIntyre, S., MacIver, S., & Sooman, A. (1993). Area, class and health: Should we be focusing on places or people? *Journal of Social Policy, 22*, 213–234.

Maimon, D., Browning, C. R., & Brooks-Gunn, J. (2010). Collective efficacy, family attachment, and urban adolescent suicide attempts. *Journal of Health and Social Behavior, 51*(3), 307 324.

March, D., Hatch, S. L., Morgan, C., Kirkbride, J. B., Bresnahan, M., Fearon, P., et al. (2008). Psychosis and place. *Epidemiologic Reviews, 30*, 84–100.

McQuarrie, M., & Marwell, N. P. (2009). The missing organizational dimension in urban sociology. *City and Community, 8*, 247–268.

Metraux, S., Caplan, J. M., Klugman, D., & Hadley, T. R. (2007). Assessing residential segregation among medicaid recipients with psychiatric disability in philadelphia. *Journal of Community Psychology, 35*(2), 239–256.

Moore, S., Bockenholt, U., Daniel, M., Frohlich, K., Kestens, Y., & Richard, L. (2011). Social capital and core network ties: A validation study of individual-level social capital measures and their association with extra- and intra-neighborhood ties, and self-rated health. *Health and Place, 17*(2), 536–544.

Murphy, J. (1994). The Stirling County Study: Then and now. *International Review of Psychiatry, 6*, 329–348.

Pearlin, L. I. (1999). The stress process revisited. In C. S. Aneshensel & J. C. Phelan (Eds.), *Handbook in the sociology of mental health* (pp. 395–415). New York: Kluwer Academic/Plenum Publishers.

Robert, S. A. (1999). Socioeconomic position and health: The independent contribution of community context. *Annual Review of Sociology, 25*, 489–516.

Robert, S. A., Cagney, K. A., & Weden, M. M. (2010). A life course approach to the study of neighborhoods and health. In C. E. Bird, P. Conrad, A. M. Fremont, & S. Timmermans (Eds.), *Handbook of Medical Sociology* (6th ed., pp. 124–143). Nashville, Tennessee: Vanderbilt University Press.

Robinson, W. S. (1950). Ecological correlations and the behavior of individuals. *American Sociological Review, 15*(3), 351–357.

Ross, C. E. (2000). Neighborhood disadvantage and adult depression. *Journal of Health and Social Behavior, 41*, 177–187.

Ross, C. E. (2011). Collective threat, trust, and the sense of personal control. *Journal of Health and Social Behavior, 52*(3), 287–296.

Ross, C. E., & Mirowsky, J. (2009). Neighborhood disorder, subjective alienation, and distress. *Journal of Health and Social Behavior, 50*(1), 49–64.

Sampson, R. J., & Byron Groves, W. (1989). Community structure and crime: Testing social disorganization theory. *American Journal of Sociology, 94*(4), 774–802.

Sampson, R. J., Morenoff, J. D., & Gannon-Rowley, T. (2002). Assessing 'neighborhood effects': Social processes and new directions in research. *Annual Review of Sociology, 28*, 443–478.

Sampson, R. J., Raudenbush, S. W., & Earls, F. (1997). Neighborhoods and violent crime: A multilevel study of collective efficacy. *Science, 277*(5328), 918–924.

Sampson, R. J., Sharkey, P., & Raudenbush, S. W. (2008). Durable effects of concentrated disadvantage on verbal ability among African-American children. *Proceedings of the National Academy of Sciences, 105*(3), 845–852.

Scheper-Hughes, Nancy. (1979). *Saints, scholars, and schizophrenics: Mental illness in rural Ireland*. Berkeley, California: University of California Press.

Schieman, S., Pearlin, L. I., & Meersman, S. C. (2006). Neighborhood disadvantage and anger among older adults: Social comparisons as effect modifiers. *Journal of Health and Social Behavior, 47*(2), 156–172.

Schroeder, C. W. (1942). Mental disorders in cities. *American Journal of Sociology, 48*(1), 40–47.

Schwartz, S. (1994). The fallacy of the ecological fallacy: The potential misuse of a concept and the consequences. *American Journal of Public Health, 84*(5), 819–824.

Segal, S. P., Baumohl, J., & Moyles', E. W. (1980). Neighborhood types and community reaction to the mentally ill: A paradox of intensity. *Journal of Health and Social Behavior, 21*(4), 345–359.

Sharkey, P. (2010). The acute effect of local homicides on children's cognitive performance. *Proceedings of the National Academy of Sciences, 107*, 11733–11738.

Sharkey, P., & Elwert, F. (2011). The legacy of disadvantage: Multigenerational neighborhood effects on cognitive ability. *American Journal of Sociology, 116*, 1934–1981.

Sharkey, P. T., Tirado-Strayer, N., Papachristos, A. V., & Cybele Raver, C. (2012). The effect of local violence on children's attention and impulse control. *American Journal of Public Health, 102*, 2287–2293.

Silver, E., Mulvey, E. P., & Swanson, J. W. (2002). Neighborhood structural characteristics and mental disorder: Faris and dunham revisited. *Social Science and Medicine, 55*, 1457–1470.

Simmel, G. (1903). The metropolis and mental life. In K. Wolfe (Ed.), *The sociology of Georg Simmel*. pp. 409–424.

Small, M. L. (2009). *Unanticipated gains: Origins of network inequality in everyday life*. New York: Oxford University Press.

Srole, L., Langner, T. S., Michael, S. T., Opler, M. K., & Rennie, Thomas A. C. (1962). *Mental health in the metropolis: The Midtown Manhattan Study* (Vol. I). New York: McGraw-Hill.

Thoits, P. A. (1995). Stress, coping, and social support: Where are we? What next? *Journal of Health and Social Behavior, 35*, 53–79. (special issue).

Turner, H. A., Shattuck, A., Hamby, S., & Finkelhor, D. (2013). Community disorder, victimization exposure, and mental health in a national sample of youth. *Journal of Health and Social Behavior, 54*, 257–274.

Turney, K., Kissane, R., & Edin, K. (2013). After Moving to Opportunity: How moving to a low-poverty neighborhood improves mental health among African American women. *Society and Mental Health, 3*, 1–21.

Vartanian, T. P., & Houser, L. (2010). The effects of childhood neighborhood conditions on self-reports of adult health. *Journal of Health and Social Behavior, 51*(3), 291–306.

Verhaeghe, P.-P., & Tampubolon, G. (2012). Individual social capital, neighbourhood deprivation, and self-rated health in England. *Social Science and Medicine, 75*(2), 349–357.

Wheaton, B., & Clarke, P. (2003). Space meets time: Integrating temporal and contextual influences on mental health in early adulthood. *American Sociological Review, 68*, 680–706.

Wilson, W. J. (1987). *The truly disadvantaged: The inner city, the underclass, and public policy.* Chicago: University of Chicago Press.

Wolch, J., & Philo, C. (2000). From distributions of deviance to definitions of difference: Past and future mental health geographies. *Health and Place, 6*(3), 137–157.

Chapter 6
Everything Old Is New Again: Recovery and Serious Mental Illness

Dennis P. Watson, Anne McCranie and Eric R. Wright

6.1 Introduction

The sociology of mental health has a long tradition of studying the social patterning of mental health, the meanings of illness and disorder, and the organization of treatment. Sociologists also have focused on the ways in which mental illness is socially constructed. However, one shift in research and policy over the past 20 years that has received relatively scant sociological attention is the concept of recovery from mental illness, particularly "serious mental illness" (SMI).

For the purposes of this paper and in keeping with the field of mental health services research, we define SMI as a mental, behavioral, or emotional disorder that meets psychiatric diagnostic criteria, which results in impairments that substantially limit an individual's major life activities such as school, work, or parenting (e.g., bipolar disorder, major depression, psychotic disorders such as schizophrenia; see President's New Freedom Commission on Mental Health 2003). A rule of thumb: all mental distress can be considered serious, but if it responds quickly and well to treatment or does not create functional impairment in a person, it is usually not

---

D.P. Watson (✉)
Indiana University Richard M. Fairbanks School of Public Health,
IUPUI, 714 N. Senate Ave, Suite EF200, Indianapolis, IN 46202, USA
e-mail: dpwatson@iu.edu

A. McCranie
Department of Sociology, Indiana University Bloomington, Bloomington, USA
e-mail: amccrani@indiana.edu

E.R. Wright
Department of Sociology, School of Public Health, Georgia State University, Atlanta, USA
e-mail: ewright28@gsu.edu

referred to as SMI. Within mental health services research, the concept of recovery is most often applied to schizophrenia and psychoses, though many researchers do not specify any particular illness.

Broadly expressed, recovery is the idea that people (most especially those diagnosed with SMI) can get better. Rehabilitation scholar Anthony has offered one of the most cited definitions:

> Recovery is a deeply personal, unique process of changing one's attitudes, values, feelings, goals, skills, and/or roles. It is a way of living a satisfying, hopeful, and contributing life even with limitations caused by illness. Recovery involves the development of new meaning and purpose in one's life as one grows beyond the catastrophic effects of mental illness (Anthony 1993: 527).

While this definition is relatively recent, it is important to understand that ideas of improvement from mental illness have circulated for generations including: the optimism of the moral treatment movement in the 19th century; the public stir caused by ex-patient Clifford Beer's advocacy in the early 20th century; and the push for community support programs beginning in the 1970s (Davidson et al. 2010).

Beyond the modest idea that recovery is about the belief that people with SMI can "get better," we do not offer a single definition of the term ourselves. Indeed, as we discuss below, the concept continues to be the subject of debate within the field. Further, and more important for sociologists, it stands to reason that as much as "mental illness" and "mental disorder" are socially constructed concepts, so too is "recovery." Like mental illness or disorder, recognizing the socially constructed nature of a problem does not mean that we are denying its reality—just as people clearly suffer from what is called disorder, so do they get better from it. Our aim in this paper is to briefly outline the history of recovery (including how it has been defined by various interest groups and how it is reflected in current practice), examine its role in the sociology of mental health and illness, and discuss the significance for future sociological work.

6.2 Cultural History of Recovery

The roots of the modern concept of recovery have been traced to Philippe Pinel who applied his ideas of *traitment moral* (i.e., moral treatment) in his work in the asylums of Paris over 200 years ago (Davidson et al. 2010). However, the idea of recovery did not take hold in popular culture or clinical work until the 1980s. This is because of pervasive historical beliefs that the course of SMI (in particular schizophrenia) was a chronic downward spiral. These negative views stemmed primarily from work conducted in the early 1900s by German psychiatrist Kraepelin ([1913] 1987) whose observations of his patients led him to the conclusion that schizophrenia, which he called *dementia praecox*, was a progressively degenerative disease. Popular associations between mental illness and dangerousness are a legacy of Kraepelin's work that served to legitimize the wide-scale institutionalization of people living with SMI in state psychiatric hospitals (Davidson 2003; Szasz [1961] 1989). For many individuals, commitment to these institutions was a life-long sentence.

A number of developments beginning in the 1950s in the United States opened up the possibility for recovery from SMI to be recognized as a legitimate possibility and the goal of mental health treatment. First, new laws (reflecting changing social values) defined patient rights—including the right not to be institutionalized—and established quality of care standards thanks to the efforts of advocates and ex-patients who worked to make the general public more aware of the dehumanizing conditions in state hospitals (Kaufmann 1999; McLean 2009). At the same time, medications were developed that were able to control some of the more difficult to manage symptoms associated with psychotic disorders (Scheid and Greenberg 2007). The need for institutional care gradually lost its legitimacy, and there were increasing calls for a community-based care system. Changing financing structures resulted in the wide-scale dismantling of state psychiatric hospitals (Mechanic and Rochefort 1990). Landmark U.S. community mental health center legislation, part of broader progressive social welfare expansion, passed in 1963 and led to the dramatic increase in the federal commitment to mental health services.

While it seems as though a focus on recovery would have been a logical part of the plan for the move to community-based care, this was not the case. There was, in short, no plan. Deinstitutionalization, a "disjointed, non-linear process" as Mechanic and Rochefort (1990: 306) call it, was the result of a confluence of events and forces. The move to a true community-based care system never became a reality, though it gained significant policy interest and inspired incremental reforms in the United States in the late 1970s and through the early 1990s (Grob and Goldman 2006).

By the time psychiatric rehabilitation researcher William Anthony published his "guiding vision" piece in 1993—a work that would go on to be the single most highly cited work in the field—there had been many other forces at play that encouraged a rhetoric of recovery. First, a number of studies resulted from the move to community-based care that demonstrated (a) the course of SMI (schizophrenia in particular) was not as predictable as once thought and (b) recovery (measured through remission of symptoms) was a reality that often occurred without any type of professional intervention (DeSisto et al. 1995; Harding 1988; Harding et al. 1987a, b, d). Second, the emergence and subsequent actions of the mental health consumer and survivor movements led to changes in the way SMI is viewed within society, as well as a number of important policy and legal developments that have greatly increased the rights of those living with a mental health diagnosis and placed greater emphasis on recovery within the treatment system (Frese and Davis 1997; McLean 2009; Jacobson 2004; Tomes 2006; Zinman et al. 1987).

6.3 Contested Views of Recovery

The historical changes discussed above demonstrate that recovery is a social construction that has been intimately tied to changes in the way mental illness has been understood over the past 200 years. While the major consensus today is that recovery can and does occur, there is still considerable disagreement over what the term actually means (Farkas 2007; Fitzpatrick 2002; Jacobson and Greenley 2001; Onken et al. 2007; Roe et al. 2007). Psychiatrists Liberman and Kopelowicz (2005) have argued that recovery can be conceptualized in one of two ways. First, there are those who define *recovery as an outcome*. Those who adhere to this perspective generally tend to measure recovery in one of three ways: (1) complete remission; (2) symptom improvement; or (3) meeting clinically predetermined goals (e.g., treatment adherence, medication compliance, etc.). Second, are those who define *recovery as a process* or journey that emphasizes factors such as empowerment, personhood, and quality of life (Anthony 1993; Corrigan and Ralph 2005). Liberman and Kopelowicz argue that this second notion should actually be more appropriately referred to as "recovering." In essence, they argue that *recovery* is a state that people might achieve; *recovering* is how they get there.

The *outcome* perspective of recovery tends to be followed to a greater degree among researchers with a more biomedical and/or psychiatric focus and the difficulty in finding a clear and definitive definition of recovery has frustrated some researchers who fit within this camp. This group argues that the idea must be tied to functional or symptomatic remission, lest it become a meaningless or even dangerous idea (Bellack 2006; Roe et al. 2007). For instance, Andreasen, a schizophrenia researcher, and a group of highly influential neurobiologically-oriented psychiatrists recently offered a set of remission criteria to be encompassed within the broader idea of recovery. In this formulation, remission is an "improvement in core signs and symptoms of mental illness to the extent that they are below a clinically diagnosable threshold and no longer interfere significantly with behavior, while recovery is the ability to function relatively free of disease in a community setting" (Andreasen et al. 2005). In this formulation, remission is a necessary part of the path to recovery, a standard some recovery-oriented researchers, policymakers, and consumer advocates would explicitly reject. This set of criteria that Andreasen and colleagues put out is the first consensus-based definition of symptomatic remission, and it has attracted a significant amount of research attention from those looking for "objective" outcomes that emphasize improvement.

The *process* perspective is more popular among advocates, policymakers, and those who espouse the goals of psychosocial rehabilitation. The United States Substance Abuse and Mental Health Services Administration (SAMHSA) recently offered a new concensus-based working definition that recovery is "[a] process of change through which individuals improve their health and wellness, live a self-directed life, and strive to reach their full potential" (2012: paragraph 5). However, the new definition does not stop there. There are four "dimensions" to recovery: *health* (where, presumably the concern with symptom reduction would be categorized), *home* (housing), *purpose* (work, education, independence) and *community* (relationships and networks), ant ten additional "guiding principles" of recovery cover both social and personal areas (e.g., need for hope, the benefit of peer relationships, the need for "person-driven" services, etc.). This definition of recovery has something for everyone, it appears.

Outcome versus process is just one contested dimension found in the recovery literature. A second and equally important debate (one that will ring familiar to sociologists) focuses on the tension between deficit and disability. Davidson and Roe (2007) make a different distinction between outcomes, that of recovery *from* versus recovery *in mental illness*. Recovery *from* is the positive outcome and is similar to what Liberman and Kopelowicz suggest. However, it is more open-ended than their formulation in that it is less focused on the objective criteria and more concerned with improvement on previous deficits. Recovery *in* mental illness reads far more like a social disability model of mental health:

> Recovery in this sense is a recovery of place in society, regardless of the functional or symptomatic conditions of a person. Recovery refers instead to overcoming the effects of being a mental patient – including poverty, substandard housing, unemployment, loss of valued social roles and identity, isolation, loss of sense of self and purpose in life, and the iatrogenic effects of involuntary treatment and hospitalisation – in order to retain, or resume, some degree of control over their own lives. (2007: 462)

So, accordingly, recovery here refers to two kinds of outcomes: one individualized and focused on correcting perceived deficits and one political and focused on correcting a disabling social structure that harms people and keeps them at disadvantage.

As we will discuss below, some of the distinctions drawn here reflect structural cleavages in the treatment of people with SMI—namely that of a lower status rehabilitation model aimed at functional improvement (even without symptomatic reduction of problems) and the other more elevated (and psychiatrically inclined) biomedical model aimed at symptomatic reduction.

6.4 How "Recovery" Is Reshaping Mental Health Care

Placing a heavy emphasis on consumer choice and empowerment, current mental health policy closely reflects the process perspective of recovery, and these policies have given rise to and legitimated a number of mental health treatment and service innovations. We discuss several such approaches below. All of them employ a *process*-based understanding of recovery, one that emphasizes the personal journey over the ultimate destination of *outcome*. This emphasis is deliberate. While outcomes-based understandings certainly reflect an increased optimism, it is the process-oriented approaches that emphasize new forms of activity and structures within the mental health treatment system.

6.4.1 Consumer Engagement Approaches

Shared decision making (SDM) is a clinical approach that emphasizes communication, sharing of information, and consensus between patient and physician. Adams and Drake (2006) argue that the field of mental health services has endorsed the idea of negotiated decision-making for decades without explicitly labeling it as "shared decision making." It is explicitly included in recovery-based treatment models today, often as part of an explicit empowerment approach (Deegan and Drake 2006).

Closely connected to SDM, illness self-management moves a step further. It refers to a set of curriculum-based approaches aimed at getting the individual to be an "active partner" in their own treatment, beyond the decision-making process. Taking place in a one-on-one or group settings, the focus in illness management and recovery (IMR)—an illness self-management program—is education on illness, treatment, coping, and skills development. Wellness Recovery and Action Plan™ (WRAP) is a widely adopted type of illness self-management developed by Copeland ([1997] 2002). It is a curriculum designed to be taught weekly by peers over approximately two months with the goal of reducing depression and anxiety and increasing an individual's coping skills and resources. While there is only a small (but growing) research literature on the outcomes of WRAP, it has become a very popular intervention in community mental health centers in the U.S., perhaps in part, because of its flexibility and that it is relatively easily billable under Medicaid.

Taking this shared decision making process a bit further, Deegan's newer (2010) "Common Ground" approach to medication co-management with psychiatrists and individuals with SMI is a web-based application that aims to empower individuals to be able to communicate more clearly about their medication and treatment concerns. Deegan's program—which walks individuals through a series of inventories about what is most important to them in their own lives and how the medication they are on might be blocking their own no-pharmaceutical "personal medicine"—can provide a direct challenge to the traditional patient-provider interaction by both enabling discussion and dissent on the part of individuals receiving treatment.

6.4.2 Social Disability Approaches

Mental health treatment and services that follow a social disability approach tend to view the root cause of impairment as society's failure to provide accommodations to facilitate social inclusion (Mulvany 2000). As such, their primary foci are social inclusion, citizenship, and human rights. Therefore, the goal of these services is the provision of resources that allow the individual to live a more full life rather than the provision of treatment.

The *Housing First Model* (*HFM*) is a strong example of this service approach. Developed in the early 1990s as an approach to housing individuals with co-occurring SMI and substance use disorder (COD), the HFM provides immediate access to housing for individuals who are chronically homeless (Tsemberis and Asmussen 1999). The primary goal of the model is housing retention, and participants do not have to engage in any mental or behavioral health treatment if they do not wish to. The theory behind the model is that symptoms and problems associated with mental illness are caused and/or exacerbated by a lack of access to basic necessities or rights. Therefore, the provision of housing is an intervention in itself that will lead to improved mental health and quality of life, among other outcomes. Indeed, the HFM has been demonstrated to lead to improvements in both housing retention over other housing models that require treatment participation and more perceived choice in services (Greenwood et al. 2005; Tsemberis et al. 2004).

The HFM's emphasis on human rights and consumer choice is reinforced in its use of *harm reduction* practices. Not unique to the HFM, harm reduction seeks to eliminate the negative consequences associated with high risk behaviors, rather than eliminating the behavior itself (Marlatt 1996). Due to its beginnings as a substance abuse intervention, harm reduction has become a popular approach for working with individuals living with CODs (see Tsemberis et al. 2004). Providers who follow this approach work to develop risk reduction plans with consumers who do not wish to take medications and/or stop using drugs. An example of this might be making sure consumers have access to condoms so that it is more likely they will engage in safe sex when their judgment is impaired.

Services that fit within a social disability framework are more realistic options for consumers who traditionally have been considered "hard-to-serve" due to the complexity or severity of their problems. For instance, individuals with CODs often have difficulty obtaining appropriate treatment because of service providers' reluctance to work with both disorders or because they have difficulty meeting program demands (e.g., sobriety, medication compliance, high levels of service engagement, etc.) due to the severity of their problems. When it is received, treatment is often provided by both systems simultaneously, which can compound problems considering there is often dissonance between the process-focused recovery goals of the mental health system and the outcome-focused (i.e., abstinence) recovery goals of the substance abuse system (Davidson and White 2007). Social disability focused services like the HFM and harm reduction have proven successful with this population because their focus on human rights and consumer choice means that they are easily accessible and have limited demands that lead to higher retention.

6.4.3 Peer Involvement in Treatment

Davidson et al. (2006) identified three main strains of peer services: mutual support, consumer-run services, and peers as providers. Involving individuals with mental health problems in the treatment and support of their "peers" is not a new concept by any means, particularly in the form of "self-help" groups. Abraham Low, a state hospital psychiatrist, for example, formed self-help groups for individuals discharged from hospitals stays in the late 1940s (Low [1943] 1991). These mutual support groups focused on self-esteem, goal-setting, and coping, and are not terribly different from the support groups offered in many modern treatment systems. "Recovery, Inc.", Low's organization and model, still exists today and has been joined by a variety of other types mutual support groups.

Peer-focused and peer-run services have evolved and expanded over the years, particularly since in the 1970s. Indeed, many such programs have become critical components of many treatment programs for people diagnosed with SMI, although these programs are generally not systematically available in all areas across the United States. The clubhouse model, popularized by Fountain House in New York City, is the most well-known psychosocial rehabilitation model of recovery. Clubhouse programs are typically organized around consumer-run programs and extensive peer-to-peer interaction. In part, because of the extensive involvement of peers, these programs are often argued by advocates and some professionals to be more truly "recovery-focused" forms of care because they are more clearly distinguishable and different from more traditional biomedical approaches to treatment.

One of the most striking developments in recent years in the United States has been the growth of programs that involve peers-as-providers (sometimes styled "peer recovery specialists"), and Medicaid has recently created a designation of "semi-professional providers" that can be used for billing purposes. Georgia was the first state to introduce peer specialist certification in 2001 and by 2012 peer specialist programs were present in 23 states (Grant et al. 2012). Reimbursement and organization of this new category of mental health professional vary widely, though education and ongoing supervision by a trained professional is a requirement. Peer specialists work within traditional behavioral health settings and are often involved in activities that providers might also be engaged with (such as illness management and recovery curriculum) or in a group treatment setting. This new "professional" category is built on the identity of being a person in recovery from a mental illness.

6.5 Sociological Contributions to Recovery Research

While only a few sociologists of mental health have paid direct attention to the topic of recovery, a number of early sociological and sociologically-oriented studies have had direct and indirect lasting effects on the recovery movement. Indeed, Goffman's 1961 essay, *The Moral Career of the Mental Patient*, was the first work to demonstrate the significant influence that the structure of care had over the course of mental illness (of which recovery is part). This work, along with a number of other sociologically-informed studies brought to light a number of problems associated with institutional treatment and helped provide legitimacy to the argument for community-based care (Hillery 1963; Lefton et al. 1959; Street 1965; Wallace and Rashkis 1959). There also now is mounting empirical evidence that symptom remission related to schizophrenia is associated with a number of sociological forces, including social class, education, and access to care (Harding et al. 1987c; Harding 1988; Robins and Regier 1991). Finally, sociological studies of the social experiences of people in psychiatric treatment also have established the powerful effects of diagnostic labeling and stigma on mental patient's lives; research that contributed powerfully to the growth of the Mental Health Survivor Movement (Scheff 1999; Szasz 1961).

Given the historical connections between sociological research and the recovery movement, why has the discipline given so little direct attention to the study of recovery? One reason is that sociologists of mental health began moving away from the studying SMI in the 1980s—the same time that epidemiological studies were providing evidence of recovery from schizophrenia—in favor of studying those with less severe problems (Mulvany 2000; Pescosolido et al. 2007). Indeed, sociologists are more likely to examine the effects that social phenomena have on mental health, rather than looking at the social consequences of mental illness, an area of inquiry more directly applicable to the study of recovery (Markowitz 2005; Pescosolido et al. 2007).

Sociologists who study stigma and labeling are clearly an exception, as the majority of work in this area is concerned with understanding the social effects—positive or negative—of mental health diagnoses and treatment (Gove 1975, 1982, 2004; Gove and Fain 1977; Link et al. 1989, 1997; Link and Phelan 2001; Phelan 2005; Rosenfield 1997; Thoits 2005; Wright et al. 2007). Indeed, Gove's (1970, 1980) work addressed what he calls the "restitutive process," a theoretical construct closely related to that of recovery. The concept of mental illness as a "career", initially intellectualized by Goffman (1961), continues to influence the theoretical thinking of many sociologists of mental health, particularly labeling theorists (see Aneshensel 2013); however, very little work in this area has focused on the processes and outcomes beyond the stages associated with diagnosis and treatment.

Sociologists also have tended to conceptualize mental health and illness as continuous variables as opposed to a discrete diagnostics status common in other disciplines (Wheaton 2001). The continuous perspective is highly compatible with the process view of recovery because it recognizes that variations in the severity of mental illness exist. Keyes's work (2002, 2007) suggests that mental health and illness exist along two separate continua and challenge the widely held views that mental health and illness are an either/or dichotomy or that they exist on separate ends of the same continuum. His findings dovetail with recovery researchers' work that demonstrates symptoms of mental illness often coexist with signs of healthy functioning during the recovery process (see Anthony 1993; Borg and Davidson 2008). Clearly, this multidimensional, continuous approach to conceptualizing and measuring mental health and illness holds significant promise for future recovery research.

On the other hand, there have been a few sociological works that have directly addressed the topic of recovery. Markowitz (2005) has contributed one of the first sociological models of recovery that draws on interdisciplinary writings; integrates such concepts as social causation and selection, social stress, and stigma; and provides concrete suggestions for future sociological recovery-focused research. He also has carried out empirical studies to test his theory and demonstrate the relevance of social factors to the recovery process. For example, using longitudinal data collected from consumers engaged in self-help and outpatient treatment, he demonstrated that economic stability and social relationships were positively related to life satisfaction and decreased mental health symptoms and provided evidence that self-concept, as it relates to recovery, is a product of social interaction (Markowitz 2001). Further highlighting the connections between social interaction and self-concept and providing additional support for modified labeling theory, Markowitz et al. (2011) found evidence that mental health symptoms and level of functioning are influenced by the perceptions of others, how mentally ill people believe others perceive them, and self-perceptions.

McCranie (2010) has argued that recovery should be considered a social movement within mental health services research that has a long history but is experiencing a current resurgence. Jacobson's (2003, 2004) work has demonstrated how recovery is a social construction that is subject to personal, professional, and political influences. In addition, Jacobson has offered a provocative theoretical framework for understanding the recovery process, a concept that proves difficult to define due to the uniqueness of each person's experience. Specifically, in an analysis of recovery narratives, Jacobson (2001) posits four central dimensions of recovery (self, others, the system, and the problem) upon which she makes recommendations for policy and practice. Jacobson also developed a conceptual model of recovery with Greenley that pragmatically links the conditions understood to facilitate recovery with the strategies, structures, and individuals that can support them (Jacobson and Greenley 2001).

Pilgrim (2008), a British sociologist, has pointed out that recovery is a "polyvalent concept" in the world of mental health policy and treatment. His research highlights how the bio-medically oriented approaches (recognizable as the "objective outcome" sense of the term) clash with the optimistic psychosocial rehabilitation model of improvement and are even more starkly contrasted with the "dissenting service user" approach. The latter takes a more social disability view of recovery and emphasizes the ways in which societal structures—particularly that of the treatment system are oppressive.

Yanos et al. (2007) developed a sociological framework that points to the importance of understanding the connections between social structure and agency as they apply to the recovery process. And,Watson (2012) applied Yanos et al.'s framework in his investigation of the impact of housing services on the mental health recovery of the formerly homeless. His analysis demonstrated the influence that service structures can have on the recovery process through their effect on an individual agency.

Finally, New Zealand sociologist Scott (2011) has explored the emotional labor required of the new semi-professional ranks of mental health workers—peer specialists. These paid providers, identified as individuals living with mental illness themselves, are engaged in assisting other individuals with their recovery. Their work, Scott argues is "authenticity work," a conundrum created by the need to be fully authentic in their professional relationships.

6.6 Conclusion: Toward a Sociology of Recovery

If there is a sociology of mental health and illness, there can and should be a sociology of recovery. Indeed, we maintain that sociologists have the potential to make significant contributions to the ongoing public, policy, and scientific debates regarding the potential for recovery from mental illness. At the micro-level, there are many outstanding questions about the meaning of recovery and how different people experience it. Prior sociological work suggests that social psychological factors, social networks and support, involvement with the treatment system, stigma, and other community conditions can shape people's understanding and perceptions of mental illness. Future work will need to examine these—and many other—factors carefully if we wish to truly understand individuals' experiences of recovery.

At the macro-level, there is growing evidence that recovery, like mental illness, is stratified (Warner 1994). Sociologists could make major contributions to the field by giving more attention to the social distribution of recovery, just as many sociologists have contributed to the extensive body of work on the social epidemiology of mental illnesses. Knowing which social groups are more or less likely to experience different types of recovery would yield important new insights on the extent and nature of disparities in recovery and foster a greater awareness and understanding of the social determinants of recovery.

At a more general level, sociologists also should examine more closely the social and historical origins and evolution of the concept of recovery itself. In this paper, we briefly examined recovery as a social construct and movement within the research field and tried to highlight the contested nature of recovery as it currently reflected within the mental health system. Our analysis underscores both the contested nature of recovery and the fact that the current debate reflects, and is deeply embedded in, competing professional conceptualizations of mental illness. Future work in this area will demand a thoughtful re-examination of our existing understanding of the socio-historical construction of mental illness and a more careful consideration of the parallel emergence of the recovery construct as an equally contested yet related paradigm.

In conclusion, the recent emergence and expanded emphasis on recovery within mental health policy and practice represents an important turning point in the long-history of societal efforts to address mental health and illness. There are many new opportunities for sociologists to examine fundamental sociological concerns as well as long-standing theoretical ideas and assumptions about mental illness. More important, we believe that by focusing more attention on the sociological dimensions of recovery and the development of a new sociology of recovery, we will ultimately contribute to a more comprehensive and robust sociology of mental health and illness.

References

Adams, J. R., & Drake, R. E. (2006). Shared decision-making and evidence-based practice. *Community Mental Health Journal, 42*, 87–105.

Andreasen, N. C., Carpenter, W. T., Kane, J. M., Lasser, R. A., Marder, S. R., & Weinberger, D. R. (2005). Remission in schizophrenia: Proposed criteria and rationale for consensus. *American Journal of Psychiatry, 162*, 441–449.

Aneshensel, C. S. (2013). Mental illness as a career: Sociological perspectives. In C. S. Aneshensel, J. C. Phelan & Alex Bierman (Eds.), *Handbook of the sociology of mental health* (2nd ed., pp. 603–620). New York: Springer.

Anthony, W. A. (1993). Recovery from mental illness: The guiding vision of the mental health service system in the 1990s. *Psychosocial Rehabilitation Journal, 16*(4), 11–23.

Bellack, A. S. (2006). Scientific and consumer models of recovery in schizophrenia: Concordance, contrasts, and implications. *Schizophrenia Bulletin, 32*, 432–442.

Borg, M., & Davidson, L. (2008). The nature of recovery as lived in everyday experience. *Journal of Mental Health, 17*, 129–140.

Copeland, M. E. ([1997] 2002). *Wellness action recovery plan*. West Dummerston, VT: Peach Press.

Corrigan, P. W., & Ralph, R. O. (2005). Introduction: Recovery as consumer vision. In R. O. Ralph & P. W. Corrigan (Eds.), *Recovery in mental illness: Broadening our understanding of wellness* (pp. 3–18). Washington: American Psychological Association.

Davidson, L. (2003). *Living outside mental illness: Qualitative studies of recovery in schizophrenia*. New York, NY: New York University Press.

Davidson, L., O'Connell, M., Tondora, J., Styron, T., & Kangas, K. (2006). The top ten concerns about recovery encountered in mental health system transformation. *Psychiatric Services, 57*(5), 640–645.

Davidson, L., Rakfeldt, J., & Strauss, J. S. (2010). *The roots of the recovery movement in psychiatry: Lessons learned*. Hoboken, NJ: Wiley-Blackwell.

Davidson, L., & Roe, D. (2007). Recovery from versus recovery in serious mental illness: One strategy for lessening confusion plaguing recovery. *Journal of Mental Health, 16*, 459–470.

Davidson, L., & White, W. (2007). The concept of recovery as an organizing principle for integrating mental health and addiction services. *The Journal of Behavioral Health Services and Research, 34*(2), 109–120.

Deegan, P. E. (2010). A web application to support recovery and shared decision making in psychiatric medication clinics. *Psychiatric Rehabilitation Journal, 34*, 23–28.

Deegan, P. E., & Drake, R. E. (2006). Shared decision making and medication management in the recovery process. *Psychiatric Services, 57*(11), 1636–1639.

DeSisto, M., Harding, C. M., McCormick, R. V., Ashikaga, T., & Brooks, G. W. (1995). The Maine and Vermont three-decade studies of serious mental illness, II: Longitudinal course comparisons. *The British Journal of Psychiatry, 167*, 338–342.

Farkas, M. (2007). The vision of recovery today: What it is and what it means for services. *World Psychiatry, 6*, 68–74.

Fitzpatrick, C. (2002). A new word in serious mental illness: Recovery. *Behavioral Healthcare Tomorrow, 11*, 16–21, 33, 44.

Frese, F. J., & Davis, W. W. (1997). The consumer-survivor movement, recovery, and consumer professionals. *Professional Psychology: Research and Practice, 28*(3), 243–245.

Goffman, E. (1961). The moral career of the mental patient. In *Asylums: Essays on the social situation of mental patients and other inmates* (pp. 125–169). New York, NY: Anchor Books.

Gove, W. R. (1970). Society reaction as an explanation of mental illness: An evaluation. *American Sociological Review, 35*(5), 873–884.

Gove, W. R. (1975). The labelling theory of mental illness: A reply to Scheff. *American Sociological Review, 40*(2), 242–248.

Gove, W. R. (1980). Labeling and mental illness: A critique. In W. R. Gove (Ed.), *The labeling of deviance: Evaluating a perspective* (2nd ed., pp. 53–97). London: Sage.

Gove, W. R. (1982). Labelling theory's explanation of mental illness: An update of recent evidence. *Deviant Behavior, 3*(4), 307–327.

Gove, W. R. (2004). The career of the mentally ill: An integration of psychiatric, labeling/social construction, and lay perspectives. *Journal of Health and Social Behavior, 45*(4), 357–375.

Gove, W. R., & Fain, T. (1977). A comparison of voluntary and committed psychiatric patients. *Archives of General Psychiatry, 34*(6), 669–676.

Grant, E. A., Daniels, A. S., Powell, I. G., Fricks, L., Goodale, L., & Bergeson, S. (2012). Creation of the pillars of peer support services transforming mental health systems of care. *International Journal of Psychosocial Rehabilitation, 16*, 22–30.

Greenwood, R. M., Schaefer-McDaniel, N. J., Winkel, G., & Tsemberis, S. J. (2005). Decreasing psychiatric symptoms by increasing choice in services for adults with histories of homelessness. *American Journal of Community Psychology, 36*, 223–238.

Grob, G. N., & Goldman, H. H. (2006). *The dilemma of mental health policy: Radical reform or incremental change?*. Piscataway, NJ: Rutgers University Press.

Harding, C. M. (1988). Course types in schizophrenia: An analysis of European and American studies. *Schizophrenia Bulletin, 14*(4), 633–643.

Harding, C. M., Brooks, G. W., Ashikaga, T., Strauss, J. S., & Breier, A. (1987a). The Vermont longitudinal study of persons with severe mental illness, I: Methodology, study sample, and overall status 32 years later. *The American Journal of Psychiatry, 144*, 718–726.

Harding, C. M., Brooks, G. W., Ashikaga, T., Strauss, J. S., & Breier, A. (1987b). The Vermont longitudinal study of persons with severe mental illness, II: Long-term outcome of subjects who retrospectively met DSM-III criteria for schizophrenia. *The American Journal of Psychiatry, 144*, 727–735.

Harding, C. M., Strauss, J. S., Hafez, H., & Lieberman, P. B. (1987c). Work and mental illness, I: Toward an integration of the rehabilitation process. *The Journal of Nervous and Mental Disease, 175*(6), 317–326.

Harding, C. M., Zubin, J., & Strauss, J. S. (1987d). Chronicity in schizophrenia: Fact, partial fact, or artifact? *Hospital & Community Psychiatry, 38*(5), 477–486.

Hillery, G. A. (1963). Villages, cities, and total institutions. *American Sociological Review, 28*(5), 779–791.

Jacobson, N. (2001). Experiencing recovery: A dimensional analysis of recovery narratives. *Psychiatric Rehabilitation Journal, 24*(3), 248.

Jacobson, N. (2003). Defining recovery: An interactionist analysis of mental health policy development, Wisconsin 1996–1999. *Qualitative Health Research, 13*(3), 378–393.

Jacobson, N. (2004). *In recovery: The making of mental health policy*. Nashville, TN: Vanderbilt University Press.

Jacobson, N., & Greenley, D. (2001). What is recovery? A conceptual model and explication. *Psychiatric Services, 52*, 482–485.

Kaufmann, C. L. (1999). An introduction to the mental health consumer movement. In A. V. Horwitz & T. L. Scheid (Eds.), *A handbook for the study of mental health: Social contexts, theories, and systems* (pp. 493–506), New York: Cambridge University Press.

Keyes, C. L. M. (2002). The mental health continuum: From languishing to flourishing in life. *Journal of Health and Social Behavior, 43*(2), 207–222.

Keyes, C. L. M. (2007). Promoting and protecting mental health as flourishing: A complementary strategy for improving national mental health. *American Psychologist, 62*(2), 95–108.

Kraepelin, E. (1913). Dementia Praecox. In J. Cutting & M. Shepherd (Eds.), *The clinical roots of the schizophrenia concept: Translations of seminal european contributions on schizophrenia* (pp. 13–24), New York, NY: Cambridge University Press.

Lefton, M., Dinitz, S., & Pasamanick, B. (1959). Decision-making in a mental hospital: Real, perceived, and ideal. *American Sociological Review, 24*(6), 822–829.

Liberman, R. P., & Kopelowicz, A. (2005). Recovery from schizophrenia: A concept in search of research. *Psychiatric Services, 56*(6), 735–742.

Link, B. G., Cullen, F. T., Struening, E., Shrout, P. E., & Dohrenwend, B. P. (1989). A modified labeling theory approach to mental disorders: An empirical assessment. *American Sociological Review, 54*(3), 400–423.

Link, B. G., & Phelan, J. C. (2001). Conceptualizing stigma. *Annual Review of Sociology, 27*(1), 363–385.

Link, B. G., Struening, E., Rahav, M., Phelan, J. C., & Nuttbrock, L. (1997). On stigma and its consequences: Evidence from a longitudinal study of men with dual diagnoses of mental illness and substance abuse. *Journal of Health and Social Behavior, 38*(2), 177–190.

Low, A. ([1943] 1991). *The techniques of self-help in psychiatric after-care*. Chicago, IL: Recovery, Inc.
Markowitz, F. E. (2001). Modeling processes in recovery from mental illness: Relationships between symptoms, life satisfaction, and self-concept. *Journal of Health and Social Behavior, 42*(1), 64–79.
Markowitz, F. E. (2005). Sociological models of recovery. In R. O. Ralph & P. W. Corrigan (Eds.), *Recovery in mental illness: Broadening our understanding of wellness* (pp. 85–99), Washington, DC: American Psychological Association.
Markowitz, F. E., Angell, B., & Greenberg, J. S. (2011). Stigma, reflected appraisals, and recovery outcomes in mental illness. *Social Psychology Quarterly, 74*(2), 144–165.
Marlatt, G. A. (1996). Harm reduction: Come as you are. *Addictive Behaviors, 21*(6), 779–788.
McCranie, A. (2010). Recovery in mental illness: The roots, meanings, and implementations of a "new" services movement. In D. Pilgrim, A. Rogers & B. A. Pescosolido (Eds.), *The SAGE handbook of mental health and illness* (pp. 471–489), London: Sage Publications.
McLean, A. (2009). The mental health consumers/survivors movement in the United States. In T. L. Scheid & T. N. Brown (Eds.), *A handbook for the study of mental health: social contexts, theories, and systems* (pp. 461–477). Cambridge, UK: Cambridge University Press.
Mechanic, D., & Rochefort, D. (1990). Deinstitutionalization: An appraisal of reform. *Annual Review of Sociology, 16*, 301–327.
Mulvany, J. (2000). Disability, impairment or illness? The relevance of the social model of disability to the study of mental disorder. *Sociology of Health & Illness, 22*(5), 582–601.
Onken, S. J., Craig, C. M., Ridgway, P., Ralph, R. O., & Cook, J. A. (2007). An analysis of the definitions and elements of recovery: A review of the literature. *Psychiatric Rehabilitation Journal, 31*, 9–22.
Pescosolido, B. A., McLeod, J. D., & Avison, W. R. (2007). Through the Looking glass: The fortunes of the sociology of mental health. In W. R. Avison, J. D. McLeod & B. A. Pescosolido (Eds.), *Mental health, social mirror* (pp. 3–32). New York, NY: Springer.
Phelan, J. C. (2005). Geneticization of deviant behavior and consequences for stigma: The case of mental illness. *Journal of Health and Social Behavior, 46*(4), 307–322.
Pilgrim, D. (2008). 'Recovery' and current mental health policy. *Chronic Illness, 4*, 295–304.
President's New Freedom Commission on Mental Health (2003). *Achieving the promise: Transforming mental health care in America*. Rockville, MD.
Robins, L. N., & Regier, A. D. (1991). *Psychiatric disorders in America: The epidemiologic catchment area study*. New York, NY: The Free Press.
Roe, D., Rudnick, A., & Gill, K. J. (2007). Commentary: The concept of "being in recovery". *Psychiatric Rehabilitation Journal, 3*, 171–173.
Rosenfield, S. (1997). Labeling mental illness: The effects of received services and perceived stigma on life satisfaction. *American Sociological Review, 62*(4), 660–672.
Scheff, T. (1999). *Being mentally ill: Sociological theory* (3rd ed.). Piscataway, NJ: Aldine Transaction.
Scheid, T. L., & Greenberg, G. (2007). An organizational analysis in the study of mental health care. In W. R. Avison, J. D. McLeod & B. A. Pescosolido (Eds.), *Mental health, social mirror* (pp. 379–405). New York, NY: Springer.
Scott, A. (2011). Authenticity work: Mutuality and boundaries in peer support. *Society and Mental Health, 1*, 173–184.
Street, D. (1965). The inmate group in custodial and treatment settings. *American Sociological Review, 30*(1), 40–55.
Substance Abuse and Mental Health Services Administration (2012). SAMHSA's working definition of recovery updated. *SAMHSA Blog*. Retrieved April 26, 2012 (http://blog.samhsa.gov/2012/03/23/defintion-of-recovery-updated/)
Szasz, T. S. (1961). *The myth of mental illness: Foundations of a theory of personal conduct*. Revised. New York, NY: Harper Perennial.
Thoits, P. A. (2005). Differential labeling of mental illness by social status: A new look at an old problem. *Journal of Health and Social Behavior, 46*(1), 102–119.

Tomes, N. (2006). The patient as a policy factor: A historical case study of the consumer/survivor movement in mental health. *Health Affairs, 25*(3), 720–729.

Tsemberis, S., & Asmussen, S. (1999). From streets to homes—The pathways to housing consumer preference supported housing model. *Alcoholism Treatment Quarterly, 17*(1), 113–131.

Tsemberis, S., Gulcur, L., & Nakae, M. (2004). Housing first, consumer choice, and harm reduction for homeless individuals with a dual diagnosis. *American Journal of Public Health, 94*(4), 651–656.

Wallace, A. F. C., & Rashkis, H. A. (1959). The relation of staff consensus to patient disturbance on mental hospital wards. *American Sociological Review, 24*(6), 829–835.

Warner, R. (1994). *Recovery from schizophrenia: Psychiatry and political economy*. London: Routledge.

Watson, D. P. (2012). From structural chaos to a model of consumer support: Understanding the roles of structure and agency in mental health recovery for the formerly homeless. *Journal of Forensic Psychology Practice, 12*(4), 325–348.

Wheaton, B. (2001). The role of sociology in the study of mental health ... and the role of mental health in the study of sociology. *Journal of Health and Social Behavior, 42*(3), 221–234.

Wright, E. R., Wright, D. E., Perry, B. L., & Foote-Ardah, C. E. (2007). Stigma and the sexual isolation of people with serious mental illness. *Social Problems, 54*(1), 78–98.

Yanos, P. T., Knight, E. L., & Roe, D. (2007). Recognizing a role for structure and agency: Integrating sociological perspectives into the study of recovery from severe mental illness. In W. R. Avison, J. D. McLeod & B. A. Pescosolido (Eds.), *Mental health, social mirror* (pp. 407–436). New York, NY: Springer.

Zinman, S., Harp, H. T., & Budd, S. (1987). *Reaching across: Mental health clients helping each other*. Riverside, CA: California Network of Mental Health Clinics.

Chapter 7
Impact of Mental Health Research in Sociology: Nearly Four Decades of Scholarship (1975–2011)

Robert J. Johnson

In the early 1980s sociology witnessed the leading crest of a wave of new and noteworthy research in the sociology of mental health that helped raise the American Sociological Association's (ASA) *Journal of Health and Social Behavior* (*JHSB*) to the highest levels of scholarly impact up to that time and later help launch a new Section of the Sociology of Mental Health. Prior to that point, research on topics of mental health were present among the founding and most influential works in both European and American Sociology as well. Today, 20 years after its formation in 1992, the Section of the Sociology of Mental Health (SSMH) is large and vibrant with its own ASA journal, *Society and Mental Health* (*SMH*).

This article looks back at a period before the formation of the Section of the Sociology of Mental Health and traces the impact and course of mental health research in select sociology publications through that period until the first issue of the journal published last year. The formation of the section 20 years ago was especially prescient in light of the Center for Disease Control's assessment that mental health is among the top ten public health challenges we will face in the 21st century, a list that followed just less than a decade later. Koplan and Fleming (2000, p. 1697) identified those ten challenges, and noted the importance of addressing the "impact of mental health" as the "second leading cause of disability and premature mortality in the United States…." The rise in the impact of social science research into the social causes and consequences of mental health problems, perhaps then, should not be so surprising. The economy of scholarship is much like that any—scholarly productivity is in response to demand and lead by innovation, both of which should figure prominently in the fields scholarly outlets.

R.J. Johnson (✉)
University of Miami, Coral Gables, USA
e-mail: rjohnson@miami.edu

But before turning to evidence of that impact in the published literature, a brief nod is given to the early foundations followed by the early history of the formation of the section.

7.1 Early Foundations of Mental Health Research in Sociology

Although a comprehensive history of mental health research in sociology has yet to be written, when it is it will surely include the works of foundational sociologists such as Durkheim (1951) and Simmel (1903), early influences such as Wirth (1931) Faris and Dunham (1939), and those who earlier influenced American Sociology itself such as James (1890, 1907). References to the early and modern history of sociological research on mental health in the U.S. (by way of its link to Medical Sociology) can be found strewn throughout Bloom's (2002) history of Medical Sociology. Continually throughout this period, as Bloom documents, mental health has been the topic of research by prominent sociologists. It has been argued that mental health research itself has found a prominent place in sociology in the last half-century, contributing greatly to the impact of sociological research (both within and across disciplinary boundaries). Sociological research with such an impact is required for the vitality of the discipline (Pescosolido and Kronenfeld 1995).

7.2 Brief History of the Formation of the Section on the Sociology of Mental Health

There were many, obvious reasons for the formation of the section. Several people, led by Jay Turner, circulated the petitions to start a section. As time for the 1990 ASA annual meeting drew near, several potential members were prepared to make a formal proposal to form the new section. The letter formally proposing to form the new section was prepared by Turner and submitted on their behalf to the Executive Committee of the ASA on July 25, 1990 (See Appendix A).

Jay Turner presided (unelected) over the organizational meetings and over the "section in formation" during the first year concluding in the first section presentation in 1992. The first elected Chair was Mechanic in 1993 and Turner was elected as the second official chair in 1994. The subsequent chairs of the section are listed in Appendix B.

The section started strong with 396 members in 1992 and grew to 423 by 1993 (see Fig. 7.1).

Except for 3 years (2001–2003) the membership has remained above 400, varying by little more than 5 %. The last membership year, 2011, provides a notable exception to this trend when the number climbed to 457 members.

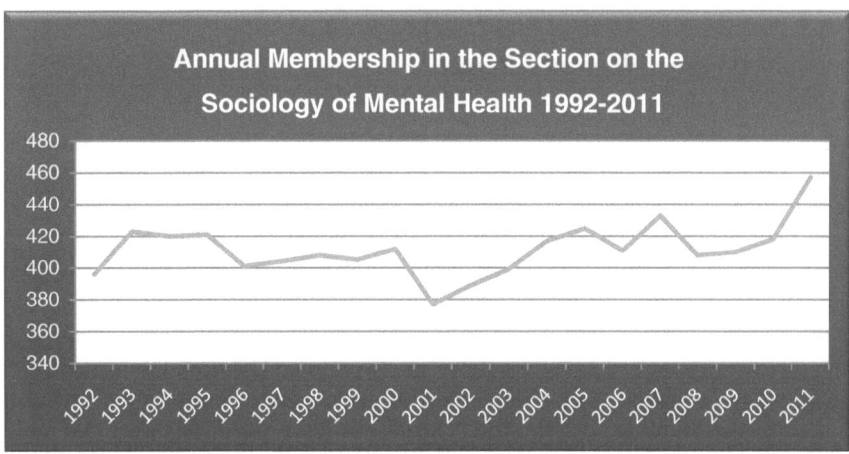

Fig. 7.1 Annual membership in the section of the sociology of mental health since its formation

7.3 Impact of Mental Health Research in Sociology

The impact of mental health research in Sociology can partially be assessed by considering the number of and citations to research articles published in the sociological literature. The data reviewed below are derived from Reuters (2012) Web of Knowledge (primarily for article counts) and Harzing (2011) Publish or Perish which uses Google Scholar (primarily for citation counts). The first database is used for article counts because it allows for convenient screening of research articles versus editorial, review, and other publication content by specific journal titles. Both databases provide similar results in terms of trends and ranks for citations.

A broad definition of mental health research that would be representative of the goals of the section would include research on particular illnesses such as anxiety or depression, more general health concerns such as stress, distress, events and trauma, reactions to stressors such as coping and social support, the social context of these including identity and status hierarchies (race, class, and gender), the social organization of mental health services, and the utilization of them. Obviously, health research more generally but also arguably nearly all sociological research have profound implications for mental health and well-being, and so the distinction between mental health research and other sociological research is a matter of overlapping boundaries (both disciplinary and interdisciplinary). Nevertheless, it is necessary to make these distinctions and in doing so, heuristics for both inclusion and exclusion are employed here.

Each publication was examined to determine whether it met the criteria for research in mental health research. Among those that did, the general topics addressed were coded to according to general topical themes that emerged during the first review. Any one article may have been coded in more than one category.

7.3.1 Sources of Mental Health Research in the Sociological Literature

The *Journal of Health and Social Behavior* (JHSB) is the primary sociological outlet for health related sociological research, being an official publication of the American Sociological Association, and thus a forum where sociologists can share their health research (including but not limited to mental health) with other sociologists. An examination of all articles appearing in the JHSB from 1975 through 2011 can provide insights not only for determining the impact of mental health research but also into trends of the sociological study of mental health during a period of time that such research was expanding (1) before the formation of the Section on Sociology of Mental Health in 1992 and (2) during the period to follow its formation. Research on the closely related topic of the legacy of stress research (though with a stated focused on stress it also included much mental health research more broadly defined here) has previously documented the rise in prominence of this journal during the earlier years of this period (Johnson and Wolinsky 1990).

Prevalence of Mental Health Research. Among the first articles found published during this period are indisputably those appearing in a special issue of JHSB in 1975 on recent developments in the "Sociology of Mental Illness." These half a dozen or so articles would be followed to eventually include 148 out of 595 research articles (excluding notes, replies, comments, or other editorial content) published through 1990. Thus nearly 25 % of all research published in the JHSB was related to the sociology of mental health. During the second period of time, 202 out of 588 research articles published in the JHSB were on the topics of mental health. This represents a substantial increase to just over one-third (34 %) of all the articles published during this period.

7.3.2 Top 100 Cited Articles in the JHSB

Prominence of Mental Health Research. Nearly two thirds of the top 100 cited article appearing between 1975 and 1990 in the JHSB were on the topic of mental health (62 %). As Fig. 7.2 shows, these earlier leading articles dealt primarily with the topics of stress, coping and social support.

The impact of these top three categories ranges from 6,000 to 12,000 citations over their lifetime (Harzing 2011). The fourth ranked category according to number of articles published that cited these dealt variously with identity, roles and social status dealt but largely with marital status, occupational status or socioeconomic status and often with multiple combinations of these. Closely following their impact was the study of life events, which often dealt with life event scales and/or the positive/negative valence associated with these events. Gender and depression ranked about evenly, and sometimes overlapped in terms of

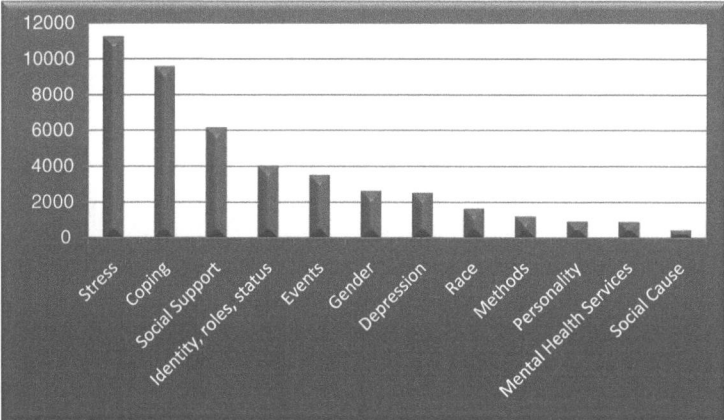

Fig. 7.2 Citations to mental health articles among the top 100 cited appearing in the JHSB 1975–1990

coverage. The former was often studied in terms of difference with the latter but certainly not always. Depression was by far the most common "disorder" used as an indicator of mental illness during this period. The study of race differences in mental health made an early appearance in the literature and certainly established itself as a palpable but not quite a leading or central theme in the sociological literature at that time. Periodically articles dealing with methodological or measurement issues would appear in this literature and while one gets the impression that they have had an impact on the direction of research in the field, that are not cited as often as substantive themes. The impact of research on mental health services appears as a theme among the top 100 cited in several articles. The appearance of personality near the end of the ranking of themes perhaps is a reflection of its "psychological" underpinnings as a topic, yet one that was still ahead of notions of purely social factors as the cause of mental illness, which appears last in this ranking. Other themes did appear from time to time, but those not listed here did not appear often among the top articles during this time period.

The second period of time (1991–2011) is reflected in Fig. 7.3 that shows citations to articles appearing in the *Journal of Health and Social Behavior*.

This period coincides with the formation and existence of the Section on Sociology of Mental Health. The number of mental health articles in the top 100 cited articles was 57 (compared to 62 earlier), a slight decline from the earlier period. Although this time period is 5 years longer, the top citation rates are lower over the lifetime of the cited articles because of the reduced exposure time (i.e., the availability of an article to be read and cited was much greater for earlier time periods than the most recent ones, a large proportion of which have only been "citable" for the last couple of years). Once again, articles that appeared in this period and primarily dealt with "stress" were having the greatest impact. However,

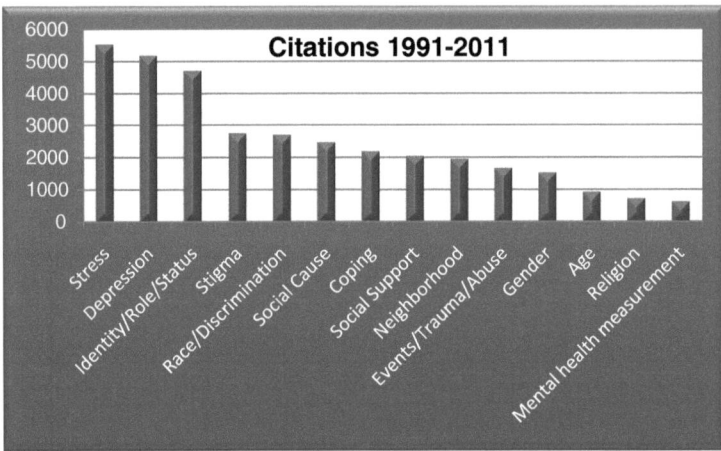

Fig. 7.3 Citations to mental health articles among the top 100 cited appearing in the JHSB 1991–2011

"coping" and "social support" slipped from ranking 2nd and 3rd to stand at 7th and 8th in the rankings of impact.

Rising to 2nd place were articles that addressed mental illness in terms of "depression" as the focal outcome, usually in combination with other themes appearing in Fig. 7.2. The themes of identity, roles, and status (while moving up only one rank) followed the 1st and 2nd ranked themes to establish a perceptively higher threshold of impact than other themes appearing during this period. The "apparent top tier" of the earlier period included primarily "stress and coping" while the "apparent top tier" during the later period included "stress" again at the top along with "depression" and "identity/roles/status." The movement of "coping" and "social support" to a second tier of influence is particularly notable. Also notable, race moved up to form the top of a 2nd tier along with the appearance of "stigma", "social cause" and "neighborhood" themes. With the upward movement of race as a theme, it had expanded to contain the effects of discrimination specifically and usually as a cause of diminished mental health (going beyond the mere documentation of racial differences in earlier research). Interestingly enough, the appearance and rise of "stigma" may be more rightly described as a "reappearance" from a body of sociological work (largely theoretical) that was popularized in earlier periods of time (i.e., labeling and dramaturgical theories of mental illness). The sociological research examining neighborhood effects on health also quickly gained strength during this period as it expanded its focus to include mental illness and other areas of social problems as well (e.g., crime). Finally, life event research endured throughout this period but it was augmented in part with a new focus on trauma and/or abuse. Gender, age, religion and measurement or methodology rounded out the impact of mental health research during this period.

Table 7.1 High impact JHSB articles by period and type

	1975–1990		1991–2011	
	Mental health	Total	Mental health	Total
JHSB 100	71 (49 %)	146	66 (52 %)	135
JHSB 500	6 (67 %)	9	5 (83 %)	6
JHSB 1000	6 (100 %)	6	2 (50 %)	4
Total	83 (52 %)	161	73 (50 %)	145

7.3.3 High Impact Articles[1]—The JHSB 100, 500, and 1,000

As the primary sociological outlet for health research in sociology, the articles published in *JHSB* have undoubtedly helped shaped the fields of medical sociology and the sociology of mental health. The citation impact for the most heavily cited articles are shown in Table 7.1. Between 1975 and 1990, 161 of the 595 articles were cited more than 100 times, 9 were cited more than 500 times, and 6 were cited more than 1,000 times. During the following period, 1991–2011, 145 of the 588 articles were cited more than 100 times, 6 were cited more than 500 times, and 4 were cited over 1,000 times. For all six categories, half or more of the high impact articles dealt with research on the topics of the sociology of mental health. During the period of 1975–1991 the mental health articles were 49 % (71 out of 146) of the JHSB 100, 67 % (6 out of 9) of the JHSB 500 and 100 % (6 out of 6) of the JHSB 1000. During the period of 1991–2011, mental health articles accounted for 49 % (66 out of 135) of the JHSB 100, 83 % (5 out of 6) of the JHSB 500 and 50 % (2 out of 4) of the JHSB 1000.

Table 7.2 refers to the 306 high impact journal articles by decade since 1975 appearing in JHSB. It often takes several years since the initial publication for high impact articles to be revealed, but between roughly the decade before and following the formation section (with a lag factor of 3-5 years) does reveal a slight decline. It is too soon and too brief a period to determine if this represents any trend.

The flagship journal of the ASA is the *American Sociological Review* (ASR) and although it is not a primary outlet for mental health related research, it remains a prominent forum for leading research to be published. The venue provides an opportunity for an examination of the impact of mental health research relative to other sociological research appearing there. The articles appearing in it from 1975 through 2011 can also provide additional insights for determining the basis of the rise in prominence of research on mental health in sociology. During the two periods under consideration, 849 (1975–1990) and 886 (1991–2011) research articles were published in the ASR. Only a small percentage during each period could be classified as mental health research according to the criteria we set above; 25 were published in the earlier period and only 11 (less than half as many) were published in the later period. The palpable decline in the number of research articles overall is even greater when considering the annual rate, 1.6 versus 0.6 per year.

---

[1] We used 100 citations as the benchmark for high impact articles following the lead of an editorial in ASR that examined the citations to articles in that journal (Jacobs 2005). The most highly cited articles (JHSB 1,000 and 500) appear in Appendix C.

Table 7.2 High impact[a] journal articles by decade since 1975

Period	Count
1975–1984	96
1985–1994	113
1995–2004	90
2005[b]	7

[a]High impact journal articles (with more than 100 citations)
[b]High impact journal articles since 2005 yet to appear

The impact of mental health research articles placed them high on the list of all articles. The large number of mental health research articles (10/25 and 6/11) were in the top 100 ASR articles published during those periods. Again, the large majority of those (15 articles during the earlier period, 10 during the latter) qualify as highly cited articles, the ASR 100 articles (Jacobs 2005) having been cited 100 times or more. The average percentile rank of these articles was at the 64th percentile (top 3rd) during 1975–1990 and at the 80th percentile (top 5th) during 1991–2011, both far above the median rank for an ASR article.

7.4 Discussion

The Section on the Sociology of Mental Health formed 20 years ago in response to a growing number of sociologists who were conducting research on mental health topics, identifying as professionals in this subspecialty, and seeking additional forums to present their scholarly work. The sociological literature published in the decades before and after the formation of the section provide evidence of what types of research was appearing and the citations to that research is evidence, in part, of the impact it was having. This evidence suggests that the surge in research in this subspecialty that was taking place was matched by prominence in scholarly impact. The prominence of this research documented for a much shorter period earlier (Johnson and Wolinsky 1990) is found here to have been present and maintained over a much broader period. This prominence was reflected in both quantity (number and proportion of articles published) and recognition (measured by citation impact) of the research appearing in the JHSB, and although the quantity palpably declined in the ASR, the recognition in terms citation impact increased from the earlier to the latter period.

These general trends over a longer period are important to note for a couple of reasons. First, citations are only a rough indication of the importance and recognition of research, especially in emerging fields that develop unevenly over shorter periods of time. The general conclusions based on the citations to the articles representing the broad subspecialty of mental health research include this range of established and developing topics of study, appearing in the same sociological journals with other sociological research having a similar range of topics. Thus, the notable features of the subspecialty as a whole over a very long period of time seem to lead to more stable conclusions. Second, while the findings on the major and minor substantive trends in mental health research itself over this period may prove to be interesting, conclusions about them must be more guarded. The emerging topics are likely to be uneven in their development, more vulnerable to short periods of obscurity or popularity. More popular research topics should not be confused with more important research topics, and neither with higher quality research. It is also true however, that seminal research should not be confused with popularity either. In terms of these data, all the research is notable because of it has been reviewed by peers and published in the leading journals of the discipline. A simple citation count after the fact is not intended to weigh (or second guess) these decisions, which after all were based on a thorough reading of each article. And to that end, we rely on editors, editorial board members and reviewers to make these judgments about what articles do and do not get published. With that in mind, we turn to examine some of the trends occurring over this period.

7.4.1 Stress

The findings show that "stress" has persisted as the most prominent topic in mental health research in Sociology. The overall early rise in prominence of mental health research (late 70s and early 80s) in the JHSB posited the putative role of the legacy of stress research itself as part of the explanation of this rise (along with other factors such as the influence of prominent stress researchers like Howard Kaplan and Leonard Pearlin serving as editors), although the distinct effect of research labeled as "stress" was not directly examined (Johnson and Wolinsky 1990). In these analyses, research labeled as "stress" did emerge as one of those distinguished topics clearly associated with the greater prominence of the research. Stress research was the most salient and persistent of all the mental health topics appearing during these years.

Near the end of the first period of analyses presented here, Pearlin (1989) wrote about the sociological study of stress in a way that both seems to sum up the previous 15 years of research evidence and predicate the following period of stress research prominence that continued during the formation and throughout the existence of the section, stating:

> Sociologists have an intellectual stake in the study of stress. It presents an excellent opportunity to observe how deeply well-being is affected by the structured arrangements of people's lives and by the repeated experiences that stem from these arrangements. Social research into stress is entirely consistent with a present-day social psychology that seeks to establish the unities between social structure and the inner functioning of individuals (House 1981a). Yet stress is not generally seen as part of a sociological mainstream, partly, I believe, because those of us who are engaged in stress research are not consistently attentive to the sociological character of the field.

In some ways, then, it does not seem like it should be any revelation that stress research should have been or remained a prominent theme in the sociological research on mental health. Stating the obvious however (even when done so by a careful, knowledgeable observer of and notable scholar in the field) often can be overlooked or even dismissed by others (who often are either less careful or knowledgeable).

7.4.2 Depression

Nearly one of two adults in the United States will experience some form of mental illness in their lifetime (Kessler et al. 2005). Major depressive disorder is among the most common mental health illnesses in the United States. Over one in five have some form of mood disorder generally and roughly one in six adults exhibit symptoms of major depressive disorder (Kessler et al. 2005). Thus it should not be surprising that it is among the most common topics of research in the sociology of mental health area.

7.4.3 Coping

The decline in the relative rank of coping research, from 2nd in the earlier period to 7th during the later period was also reflective of an absolute drop in the ratio of citations to the leading category of stress research (f_{coping}/f_{stress}). The earlier period shows coping at a ratio of 0.85 of the top cited category, while during the period following the formation of the section its ratio of 0.40 was less than half that number. What happened to coping research? Did it decline overall? If not, where did it go? The observation that coping and social support seemed to move down the impact rankings in tandem might suggest that there are similar explanations for changes in both. It makes sense, then, to turn next to the topic of social support and consider what those explanations might be. But before doing that I have a few final thoughts. As much as I suspect that the research on coping has the same characteristics that allow for a similar explanation about its relative decline, there is at the same time something unique and perhaps more psychological about it than social support. They are similar in that coping may involve the use of social support resources, and in fact, some coping strategy terminology may have morphed into social support terminology because of this overlap. Coping may also be perceived as having a greater affinity with social psychology because it is readily adapted to the clinical experience that may focus more intensely on the individual patient. As social support research moves to more closely embrace the social causes of mental illness paradigms, such a focus on individual patients and coping efforts becomes more problematic as coping can be viewed as shifting the burden to (i.e., blaming) the victim. This makes it less popular in many sociological circles.

7.4.4 Social Support

One trend that seems particularly salient for a sociological audience is the role of social support as a topic in mental health research. There is a general consensus that social support was evident in the very foundations of the sociology of mental health, and abundant evidence that it was present in an important way during the rise to prominence from the seventies into the eighties of the last century. It seems obvious that it continue to be viewed as important well through the end of the second period of impact that has been examined here a evidenced by recent attention in the prominent sociological outlets. So then why did *the relative impact* of this topic as measured by citations decline in the premier journal of the sociological study of mental health? The absolute decline in the ratio of social support impact to the leading category of stress research ($f_{social\ support}/f_{stress}$) can be readily seen by comparing Figs. 7.2 and 7.3. In this case, it declines from 0.55 to 0.37. This seems to be an especially important question in light of the evidence that shows the number of papers published in the social science literature as a whole on topics of social support went from 1,062 during the first period to 26,154 during the second period of time. Possible answers include (a) research on social support moved to other journals, primarily psychology and psychiatry, (b) the research became applicable to clinical and other professional settings and proliferated in that literature, (c) there were barriers to publishing this research in sociological literature.

In terms of where research on social support and coping is published, it has been the case that most of it has always appeared in journals other than purely sociological ones. The simple fact of the matter is that there are far more sociologists publishing in these fields than there is space in the sociological journals to include their work. The very interdisciplinary nature of mental health research from the beginning meant that sociologists would not only likely find outlets for their work in other disciplinary fields, but that sociological research on the topic would compete with and hopefully contribute to the broader interests of scholars in our own and other disciplines. Because the influence of social support on mental health is primarily a sociological phenomenon, the field of sociology in general runs the risk of not profiting more mightily from the impact and significance of this research when those sociologists can find room for their work more and more exclusively in other outlets. Ironically, however, the prestige of the discipline of sociology is enhanced across disciplines as the fruit of from its own subfield of mental health research is disseminated elsewhere. It is possible, and in fact desirable, for sociology to benefit by both taking into account the mental health research on social support in our own general studies and deriving prestige from making an impact across disciplines. My sense is that the members of the SSMH are willing and in fact anxious to do so, ever hopeful of finding a receptive audience.

7.4.5 Identity, Roles and Status

The central concept of the social self and its relationship to others in the hierarchy of society is fundamental to American Sociology arising from its earliest roots in the Chicago School. It was central through the impact that James (1890) had on the earliest introduction of pragmatism as it emerged in its central treatment by Mead (1934). James had been keenly interested in the self as a central idea in understanding mental illness, although Mead did not at least in his writings and lectures that survived. A reworking of his theories of the self, I, and me have been relevant in later critical assessments of the relationships between the mind and society. It re-emerged in the mental health research of sociologists in at least three forms: (1) the self as a psychosocial resource (self-esteem and self-mastery), (2) through its reworking by the symbolic interactionists who focus on the relationship between structure and personality through the concepts of identity, roles and status, and (3) as found in the development of social constructionism, labeling and stigma which are theoretically built on the idea of the self as socially constructed (as is expectedly mental illness as well). In its first form, the reflexive and evaluative dimension of self is viewed largely as a personal resource that might provide a salutogenic independent effect, moderating or mediating (resource depletion) response to life stressors by alleviating symptoms of distress (e.g., depression). In its second form, the sociological social psychologists also reworked the self into an examination of the structured positions of status and identity assigned to gender, race and ethnicity primarily, but as we have also seen in the findings above, in work and family. Among these most of the research in the sociology of mental health has involved gender, marital and occupational roles. In its third form, the self embodies behavioral, physical and mental illness as potentially stigmatized identities.

7.4.6 Conclusions

The scholarly field of the sociology of mental health is itself healthy and robust. Based on its foundation at the very inception of the field, its notable early history in sociology, its strong resurgence in the score of years preceding the formal organization of the SSMH, and its continuing strength in the score of years that followed, the stature of the field within the discipline is unmistakably high. The articles on mental health that appear in our flagship journal, *ASR,* are generally well cited and rank high among their peers. The same can be said for the articles that appear on mental health in the leading health journal of our field, *JHSB.* Stress research, among the many mental health topics and despite (or because) of all that has been said about it over the years, remains the frontrunner in terms of citation impact.

The earlier contributions of sociological research on stress coupled with the closely ranked impacts of coping and social support, written by sociologists appears not solely in the main sociological journals as research of high impact as noted above, but also in journals across disciplinary boundaries (psychology, psychiatry, medicine, etc.) and in interdisciplinary journals (epidemiology, public health, gerontology, human development, etc.) Evidence suggests that this research is of high enough quality to compete for journal space in and across these disciplinary boundaries and that it has high impact there as well. Perhaps one of the more revealing pieces of evidence beyond citation impact is the recent inclusion of sociological content by the Association of American Medical Colleges (2012) in the new 2015 Medical College Admissions Test (MCAT). The addition of the social and behavioral sciences in the exam was done in recognition of the impact that social factors have on health. This recognition undoubtedly comes from the years of research published by social scientists on these topics.

The reader needs only to browse the foundational topics, the "big ideas" in the MCAT preview guide (e.g., social processes, self-identity, social interaction, social structure, social inequality), to get a sense of the sociological contributions that the impact of this research has had on the field. To be sure, research on the sociology of health in general and mental health in particular is not solely responsible for this recognition that is to be shared with psychology, anthropology and other social sciences. Further analyses of citation patterns of these various topics in leading disciplinary and interdisciplinary fields outside of the sociological literature would be necessary to understand completely the relative contributions of each. However, the relative high rank of mental health research in sociology is a solid clue that the importance of its impact is secure.

There are several questions remaining about the course and impact of mental health research in sociology that might also be the focus of future research. As noted above the impact of coping and social support declined in the premier journal for sociological study of mental health. This is an especially important question because the number of papers published on topics of coping and social support increased dramatically in the social science literature. Also note that a recent update (trends and future) article by Peggy Thoits (2011) in *JHSB* had very few recent references to social support and coping from the sociological literature. This provides more evidence that leading edge research is going elsewhere than sociology. Why hasn't life course research appeared yet? Perhaps it (a) has taken hold in aging literature that doesn't move easily into the disciplinary boundaries of sociology, (b) appears only in marital and occupational transitions, (c) is perceived to have other specialized or even interdisciplinary outlets (e.g., criminology, gerontology, human development) and thus reviewers turn these manuscripts down and refer them elsewhere.

Where had stigma gone and why did it reappear? The answer to the second part of this question is easier than it is to the first. Appearing throughout the two decades that followed the formation of the SSMH were several research articles on stigma that were cited more than 100 times each. And only 3 of the 26 articles on stigma that appeared in *JHSB* were published in the period before the formation of the section. Research focusing on the impact of stigma during both periods that include other disciplines and interdisciplinary outlets would be necessary to fully answer the first part of this question. Looking at articles published in JHSB during the period following the formation of SSMH provides mixed evidence implicating several possible explanations.

7.4.7 Why Did Stress Remain Strong While Social Support and Coping Declined?

Depression remains the dominant illness outcome in the sociology of mental health research. The high prevalence of the clinical cases of depression and the dreadful scope of it as a common human experience are perhaps two of the reasons why it remains dominant as an outcome in social science research on mental health. It is a characteristic of both individual human suffering and collective social problems. In addition, sociological researchers on health topics, especially mental health topics, have long struggled with the forces exerted by the strained dichotomy of the "sociology of medicine" and the "sociology in medicine" first described by Straus (1957). This strain fosters research on both sides of the question of depression (clinical and applied on one, social construction and control on the other). Both perspectives engage in the active pursuit of scholarly activity because each concedes its significance (even if only from their own perspectives). The widespread availability of reliable and valid standardized scales, both long and short versions, in addition to the widespread acceptance of both subjective and clinical understandings of depression, is undoubtedly another reason.

Why have identity/roles/status persisted, how has this focus changed or is changing? (socioeconomic status now seems to be moving to include dimensions of wealth and other accumulated resources, or would these be better conceptualized as coping resources, or do the two lines of thought need to be integrated, or are psychosocial and economic resources a new area that needs to be explored leaving coping to types of behavior).

Are social cause, neighborhood, events, trauma and abuse related/overlapping sociological concepts? Or, if this question can be asked perhaps more appropriately in the affirmative, how are they related and where do they overlap?

What happened to gender? Is this now an area of settled findings? Or is it being marginalized again? The chapter by Simon suggests that gender and mental health is a "field of continuities and new developments." It appears that the interest in and the findings on gender may continue to be as important yet fluid as the construct itself. And even as this is being written, new challenges to the old continuities and questions about the earlier findings continue to evolve (e.g., Hill and Needham 2013).

These conclusions and further questions are necessarily more tentative than definitive, more suggestive than exhaustive as explanations for the findings or processes that produced them. The data were drawn from only two sources of sociological research, albeit those representing the flagship and leading outlets for the discipline with respect to the sociological research on mental health.

7.4.8 Caveats

As noted in the discussion above, none of our conclusions based on these findings are intended to convey meaning about the quality of one particular scholarly publication. As I indicated then, and repeated here, the intellectual and scholarly contribution made by any one journal article is still determined at the time of publication by the editors and peer reviewers of the journal. Nevertheless, there is nothing inconsistent with that in the use of citation counts to gauge the impact of a general body of scholarly work. As Garfield (1998) noted following his 1962 meeting with

Robert Merton, "The Mertonian description of normal science describes citations as the currency of science. Scientists make payments, in the form of citations, to their preceptors. Referees are supposed to help keep that Mertonian principle alive and honest." Thus in a Mertonian sense, the cumulative impact count of articles within specific areas represents a general sense of the robustness of its overall scholarly "economy" in the field. Whether or not we should be trading with this "currency" in that "economy" is another, to be sure related, topic. The restriction of these analyses to a single discipline (even further to only two journals in that discipline published by its official national association), the use of relative rankings not simply counts, and the use of such data over long periods of time help mute many of the criticisms (not all of course and perhaps silencing none completely). The reader should be aware of the intent of the analyses in light of these criticisms.

Appendix A: Text of Petition to Form the Section on the Sociology of Mental Health

University of Toronto

DEPARTMENT OF SOCIOLOGY
203 COLLEGE STREET. SUITE 301
TORONTO MST 1 P9
25 July 1990
Executive Office
American Sociological Association
1722 N Street, NW
Washington DC 20036
Dear Colleagues:

In accordance with the procedure specified in the Manual on Sections, this letter is to inform you of our intention to form a new ASA section. The section we propose is the *Sociology of Mental Health*. This section is proposed for much the same reasons that sections were originally created within the association—to promote and ensure interaction, collaboration and the exchange of concepts, research methods and scientific findings between persons of similar scholarly and/or applied interests.

The study of the social determinants of mental health and illness and of associated service providers and systems has long been recognized as a relatively distinct subject and often accorded separate treatment within social problems and other texts. The widespread recognition that there are advantages with respect to communication, service and scientific progress in viewing mental health as a distinct sub area is most clearly expressed in the administrative structure of governmental agencies. That there is a National Institute of Mental Health and departments of mental health at both state and county levels is sufficient to illustrate this point.

Sociologists in the mental health area, of course, share many interests with other medical sociologists just as medical sociologists share many interests with sociologists in the areas of deviance, organizations, etc. However, the study of health related issues has grown in size and complexity to the point where the medical sociology section is, by several hundred members, the largest in the ASA. Within such a large group there are competing interests and, indeed, ideologies that are difficult to consistently serve well year after year. We wish to emphasise that we see the proposed section as in no way a challenge to, or in competition with, the medical sociology section. Rather, we see the general area of medical sociology as so large and so diverse that it is time to institutionalize a significant aspect of this diversity.

Mental health scholars and researchers represent a significant minority of the 1,100 or so members of the medical sociology section and, we believe, account for a not insignificant fraction of the grants received and field research conducted by all sociologists in North America. We strongly feel that it is crucial for the future of our sub-area that the Association afford us a reliable opportunity to share our ideas, our work and our conclusions with one another. A separate section would achieve this goal through entitlement to sessions at our annual meeting. We have no doubt of our capacity to generate a section membership well in excess of the minimum required for a section and we urge the Committee on Sections and the Council to respond favourably to this petition.

Signed:

Appendix B: Chairs of the Section of Sociology of Mental Health

1992 R. Jay Turner (in formation)
1993 David Mechanic
1994 R. Jay Turner
1995 Leonard Pearlin
1996 Carol Aneshensel
1997 Bruce Link
1998 Mary Clare Lennon
1999 William R. Avison
2000 Sarah Rosenfield
2001 Allan V. Horwitz

2002 Nan Lin
2003 Blair Wheaton
2004 Jane D. McLeod
2005 William W. Eaton
2006 Bernice A. Pescosolido
2007 Debra Umberson
2008 Linda George
2009 Mark Tausig
2010 Heather Turner
2011 Michael Hughes
2012 Teresa Scheid
2013 Virginia Aldige Hiday

Appendix C: The JHSB 1000+ and 500+: Articles Cited 1000+ or 500+ Times Since Publication Thru 2010

Period	Author(s)	Title	Year
The JHSB 1000+			
1975–1990	Leonard I. Pearlin and Carmi Schooler	The structure of coping	1978
	Sheldon Cohen, Tom Kamarck and Robin Mermelstein	A global measure of perceived stress	1983
	Susan Folkman and Richard S. Lazarus	An analysis of coping in a middle-aged community sample	1980
	Leonard I. Pearlin, Elizabeth G. Menaghan, Morton A. Lieberman and Joseph T. Mullan	The stress process	1981
	Leonard I. Pearlin	The sociological study of stress	1989
	Peggy A. Thoits	Conceptual, methodological, and theoretical problems in studying social support as a buffer against life stress	1982
1991–2011	Peggy A. Thoits	Stress, coping, and social support processes: where are we? What next?	1995
	Bruce G. Link and Jo Phelan	Social conditions as fundamental causes of disease	1995
	Ellen L. Idler and Yael Benyamini	Self-rated health and mortality: a review of twenty-seven community studies	1997
	Ronald M. Andersen	Revisiting the behavioral model and access to medical care: does it matter?	1995
The JHSB 500+			

(continued)

Appendix C (continued)

Period	Author(s)	Title	Year
1975–1990	Barbara Snell Dohrenwend, Alexander R. Askenasy, Larry Krasnoff and Bruce P. Dohrenwend	Exemplification of a method for scaling life events: the PERI life events scale	1978
	Elaine Wethington and Ronald C. Kessler	Perceived support, received support, and adjustment to stressful life events	1986
	James M. LaRocco, James S. House and John R.P. French, Jr.	Social support, occupational stress, and health	1980
	Susan Gore	The effect of social support in moderating the health consequences of unemployment	1978
	Nan Lin, Walter M. Ensel, Ronald S. Simeone and Wen Kuo	Social support, stressful life events, and illness: a model and an empirical test	1979
	M. Audrey Burnam, Richard L. Hough, Marvin Karno, Javier I. Escobar and Cynthia A. Telles	Acculturation and lifetime prevalence of psychiatric disorders among Mexican Americans in Los Angeles	1987
	Lois M. Verbrugge	Gender and health: an update on hypotheses and evidence	1985
	Debra Umberson	Family status and health behaviors: social control as a dimension of social integration	1987
	Lois M. Verbrugge	The twain meet: empirical explanations of sex differences in health and mortality	1989
1991–2011	Ronald C. Kessler, Kristin D. Mickelson and David R. Williams	The prevalence, distribution, and mental health correlates of perceived discrimination in the United States	1999
	Christopher G. Ellison	Religious involvement and subjective well-being	1991
	Carol S. Aneshensel and Clea A. Sucoff	The neighborhood context of adolescent mental health	1996
	Ilan H. Meyer	Minority stress and mental health in gay men	1995
	James S. House, James M. Lepkowski, Ann M. Kinney, Richard P. Mero, Ronald C. Kessler, A. Regula Herzog *Source* Journal of Health	The social stratification of aging and health	1994
	Bruce G. Link, Elmer L. Struening, Michael Rahav, Jo C. Phelan, Larry Nuttbrock	On stigma and its consequences: evidence from a longitudinal study of men with dual diagnoses of mental illness and substance abuse	1997

References

AAMC (2012). MCAT^{2015}: A better test for tomorrow's doctors. Preview guide for the MCAT^{2015} exam, (2nd ed.). Association of American Medical Colleges, www.aamc.org/mcat2015

Avison, W. R., Aneshensel, C. S., Schieman, S., & Wheaton, B. (Eds.). (2010). *Advances in the conceptualization of the stress process: Essays in honor of Leonard I. Pearlin*. New York: Springer.

Bloom, S. (2002). *The word as scalpel*. Oxford: Oxford University Press.

Durkheim, E. (1951). *Suicide: A study in sociology*. New York: Free Press.

Faris, R. E. L., & Dunham, H. W. (1939). *Mental disease in urban areas*. Chicago: University of Chicago Press.

Garfield, E. (1998, May 4). The use of journal impact factors and citation analysis for evaluation of science. In *Presented at the 41st annual meeting of the council of biology editors*, Salt Lake City, UT.

Harzing, A. W. (2011). Publish or Perish 3.5. Retrieved January 2011 from http://www.harzing.com

Hill, T. D., & Needham, B. L. (2013). Rethinking gender and mental health: A critical analysis of three propositions. *Social Science and Medicine, 92*, 83–91.

Jacobs, J. (2005). ASR's greatest hits—Editor's comment. *American Sociological Review*.

William, J. (1890). The Hidden Self. *Scribner's Magazine, 7*(3).

James, W. (1907). *Pragmatism*. New York: Longmans, Green, and Co.

Johnson, R. J., & Wolinsky, F. D. (1990). The legacy of stress research: Course and impact of this journal. *Journal of Health and Social Behavior, 31*(3), 217–225.

Kessler, R. C., Berglund, P. A., Demler, O., Jin, R., & Walters, E. E. (2005). Lifetime prevalence and age-of-onset distributions of DSM-IV disorders in the National Comorbidity Survey Replication (NCS-R). *Archives of General Psychiatry, 62*(6), 593–602.

Koplan, J. P., & Fleming, D. W. (2000). Current and future public health challenges. *Journal of the American Medical Association, 284*(13), 1696–1698.

Mead, G. H. (1934). *Mind, self, and society*. Chicago, IL: The University of Chicago Press.

Pearlin, L. (1989). The sociological study of stress. *Journal of Health and Social Behavior, 30*(3), 241–256.

Pescosolido, B. A., & Kronenfeld, J. J. (1995). Health, illness, and healing in an uncertain era: Challenges from and for medical sociology. *Journal of Health and Social Behavior* (Extra Issue), 5–33.

Simmel, G. (1903). The metropolis and mental life. In K. H. Wolff (ed.) (1950), *The sociology of Georg Simmel*. New York: Free Press.

Straus, R. (1957). The nature and status of medical sociology. *American Sociological Review, 22*(2), 200–204.

Thoits, P. (2011). Mechanisms linking social ties and support to physical and mental health. *Journal of Health and Social Behavior, 52*(2), 145–161.

Reuters, T. (2012). *Web of knowledge-social science citation index (SSCI)*. New York: Thompson Reuters. (retrieved January).

Wirth, L. (1931). Clinical sociology. *American Journal of Sociology, 37*(1), 49–66.

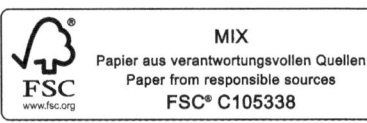

If you have any concerns about our products,
you can contact us on
ProductSafety@springernature.com

In case Publisher is established outside the EU,
the EU authorized representative is:
**Springer Nature Customer Service Center GmbH
Europaplatz 3, 69115 Heidelberg, Germany**

Printed by Libri Plureos GmbH
in Hamburg, Germany